PARASITIC DISEASES - SCHISTOSOMIASIS

Edited by **Rashika El Ridi**

Parasitic Diseases - Schistosomiasis
http://dx.doi.org/10.5772/55787
Edited by Rashika El Ridi

Contributors

Ricardo J.P.S. Guimarães, Corina Freitas, Luciano Vieira Dutra, Guilherme Oliveira, Omar Carvalho, Maria José Conceição, José Rodrigues Coura, André Ricardo Ribas Freitas, Rodrigo Nogueira Angerami, Idowu Sule Akande, Monday Francis Useh, Rashika El Ridi, Nguessan, Orsot Niangoran Mathieu, Claudineide Oliveira, Rosimeire Oliveira, Tarsila Frezza, Vera Lucia Garcia Rehder, Silmara Nascimento Fernandes De Allegretti, Denise Silveira-Lemos, Matheus Fernandes Costa Silva, Amanda Cardoso De O. Silveira, Olindo Assis Martins-Filho, Giovanni Gazzinelli, Pedro Henrique Guimarães Gazzinelli, Helena Barbosa Ferraz, Maria Carolina Barbosa Álvares, Cristiano Lara Massara, Martin Johannes Enk, Paulo Marcos Zech Coelho, Rodrigo Corrêa-Oliveira, Andréa Teixeira-Carvalho

Published by InTech

Janeza Trdine 9, 51000 Rijeka, Croatia

Copyright © 2013 InTech

Notice

Publishing Process Manager Oliver Kurelic
Technical Editor InTech DTP team
Cover InTech Design team

Additional hard copies can be obtained from orders@intechopen.com

Parasitic Diseases - Schistosomiasis, Edited by Rashika El Ridi
p. cm.
ISBN 978-953-51-0942-6

For EU product safety concerns:
IN TECH d.o.o., Prolaz Marije Krucifikse Kozulić 3, 51000 Rijeka, Croatia,
info@intechopen.com or visit our website at intechopen.com.

Meet the editor

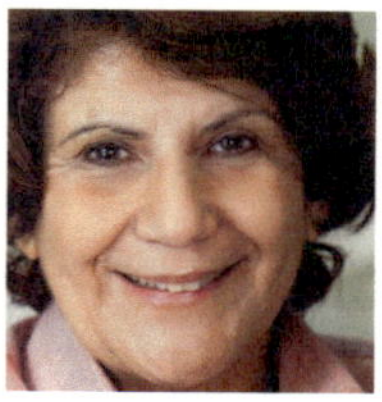

Rashika El Ridi, PhD, DSc, Professor of Immunology, Faculty of Science, Cairo University, dedicated to schistosomiasis control via development of an effective and safe drug and vaccine.

Contents

Preface

Schistosomiasis is a major public health problem in 76 countries of the developing world, yet information on prevalence and risk maps is incomplete, and often contradictory. To correct this caveat, Ricardo J.P.S. Guimarães et al. created a Geographic Information System (GIS) database, containing all social and socieconomic factors, and environmental variables, such as snail distribution, vegetation index, precipitation, temperature, and sanitation, at small communities and city levels in the Minas Gerais State, Brazil. The database was used together with multiple linear regressions to estimate the schistosomiasis positivity index, and build a schistosomiasis risk map for Minas Gerais State. The methodology used in this study can be utilized to control schistosomiasis in the areas with occurrence of the disease, and can also be used to take preventive measures to decrease or eradicate the disease transmission.

Akande and Odetola relied on community-based pilot control trials for obtaining correct and accurate estimates of schistosomiasis prevalence in Ethiopia, Tanzania, and Nigeria. Monday Francis Useh, in his chapter: Schistosomiasis, specifically reported that Schistosoma haematobium and Schistosoma mansoni infections have been widely detected in all parts of Nigeria although the former predominates. A total of 30 million Nigerians, 18% of 162 millions population, are infected with schistosomiasis, with the school age children carying the greatest burden of the disease. Of note, infection with S. haematobium was reported in all the regions in Nigeria with a prevalence as high as 60-75% among schoolchildren in some communities. N'Guessan Aya Nicaise proposed lasting solutions for fighting schistosomiasis in the Cote d'Ivoire, where urinary schistosomiasis, and soil-transmitted helminthiasis (especially hookworms), which infect > 50% of the population, prevail. The study was conducted in epidemiological context of large dam in Côte-d'Ivoire, in Taabo-village, a hyperendemic schistosomiasis locality located near Lake of the great dam Taabo, with prevalence of urinary schistosomiasis among school children reaching 94% at the start of the study. Awareness campaigns and treatments were carried out by the school teachers and Community health workers. Sociological surveys were made before treatment to understand risk behaviors. Nevertheless, slight reduction in prevalence to 74% was obtained, likely due to continuous transmission of the parasite. It was noteworthy that there was no enthusiasm for the treatment, for the simple reason that these parasites are considered by the majority of the population as non-serious illnesses and less dreadful.

The Chapters in the section "Clinical Schistosomiasis" are thus timely elaborating on the dangers not only of chronic, but also of acute schistosomiasis. According to Matheus Fernandes Costa-Silva et al., the clinical findings most commonly observed in acute schistosomiasis patients include fever, general weakness, headache, nausea, vomiting, diarrhea, anorexia, colic, weight loss, dry cough and hepatosplenomegaly accompanied by a marked eosinophilia and leucocytosis. Additionally, acute schistosomiasis is difficult to diagnose, as the clinical findings may be confounded with a number of infections such as visceral leishmaniasis, typhoid fever, malaria, tuberculosis, viral hepatitis, mononucleosis and bacterial infections. Chronic schistosomiasis mansoni and haematobium are certainly even more dangerous because of their deleterious effects on the liver, intestine, and/or urinary bladder, and additionally may involve the spinal cord, leading to neuroschistosomiasis, as documented by André Ricardo Ribas Freitas and Rodrigo Nogueira Angerami. The proportion of patients who go from schistosomiasis to medullar neuroschistosomiasis is unknown. There are several indications that this disease has been under-diagnosed, and difficult to diagnose. This situation has been changing in the last years, particularly in Brazil, due to the improvement in diagnostic tools and increase of cases in patients of of endemic countries. Finally, chronic infection with schistosomes increases the patient susceptibility to infection with viruses, namely hepatitis B and C viruses as reported by Maria Jose´Conceição and José Rodrigues Coura in the last Chapter of this section.

Accordingly, the Chapters included in the section "Drugs and Vaccines" are most welcome. Praziquantel is essentially the only drug commercially available and widely used for treatment of schistosomiasis mansoni, haematobium, and japonica. Claudineide Nascimento Fernandes de Oliveira et al. reviewed both the clinical plants that may display schistosomicidal activity and the schistosomes tegument structure, and found that fractions of plants belonging to the genus Phyllanthus L have powerful schistosomicidal effects via destruction of the tegument. The tegument lesions were thoroughly described using modified scanning and transmission electron microscopy techniques. In the last chapter of the book, Rashika El Ridi and Hatem Tallima proposed arachidonic acid as effective remedy against schistosomiasis mansoni and haematobium. The mechanism of action is likely the activation of parasite tegument associated neutral sphingomyelinase, hydrolysis of apical membrane sphingomyelin, and perturbations of the outer lipid bilayer, allowing access of host antibodies, destruction of the tegument, and eventual worm attrition. They further reported that several dogmas hinder the development of an effective vaccine, and provided rationale and evidence for the efficacy of a vaccine based on larval excretory-secretory products and Type 2 cytokines, such as interleukin-25 and 33, as adjuvants.

The chapters of this book are intended to provide useful information and strong initiative for researchers and clinicians in the field of schistosomiasis and other parasitic diseases.

At the end I wish to thank InTech, particularly Mrs. Ivona Lovric and Mr. Oliver Kurelic, for the opportunity to edit this interesting, important, and timely book, which I dedicate to the Martyrs of the Arab Spring Revolution, and to schistosome-infected children worldwide.

Rashika El Ridi
Zoology Department,
Faculty of Science,
Cairo University,
Cairo, Egypt

Section 1

Epidemiology

Chapter 1

Multiple Regression for the Schistosomiasis Positivity Index Estimates in the Minas Gerais State - Brazil at Small Communities and Cities Levels

Ricardo J.P.S. Guimarães, Corina C. Freitas,
Luciano V. Dutra, Guilherme Oliveira and
Omar S. Carvalho

Additional information is available at the end of the chapter

http://dx.doi.org/10.5772/53500

1. Introduction

Schistosomiasis, caused by *Schistosoma mansoni*, is an endemic disease conditional on the presence of snails of aquatic habits of the genus *Biomphalaria*.

In Brazil, there are eleven species and one subspecies of *Biomphalaria* genus mollusks that have been identified: *B. glabrata* (Say, 1818), *B. tenagophila* (Orbigny, 1835), *B. straminea* (Dunker, 1848), *B. peregrina* (Orbigny, 1835), *B. schrammi* (Crosse, 1864), *B. kuhniana* (Clessin, 1883), *B. intermedia* (Paraense & Deslandes 1962), *B. amazonica* (Paraense 1966), *B. oligoza* (Paraense 1974), *B. occidentalis* (Paraense 1981), *B. cousini* (Paraense, 1966) and *B. tenagophila guaibensis* (Paraense 1984) [1].

In Minas Gerais state, the presence of seven species: *B. straminea*, *B. tenagophila*, *B. peregrina*, *B. schrammi*, *B. intermedia* and *B. occidentalis* was reported [1]. Among these, there are three *Biomphalaria* species (*B. glabrata*, *B. tenagophila* and *B. straminea*) that have been found to be naturally infected with *S. mansoni*. Other three species, *B. amazonica*, *B. peregrina* and *B. cousini*, were experimentally infected, being considered as potential hosts of this trematode [2-4]. *B. glabrata* is of great importance, due to its extensive geographic distribution, high infection indices and efficiency in the schistosomiasis transmission. In endemic areas, large concentrations of these snails, together with other risk factors, favor the existence of localities with high prevalence [5-7].

The snails of the *Biomphalaria* genus live in a wide range of habitats, particularly in shallow and slow running waters and with floating or rooted vegetation. As these snails are distributed over large geographic areas and their populations are adapted to different environmental conditions, they can tolerate large variations in physical, chemical and biological environment in which they live [8, 9].

The intermediate hosts' distribution of the parasite in Minas Gerais associated with favorable eco-epidemiological conditions gives the schistosomiasis expansive character not seen even in non-endemic regions [6, 10, 11].

Public health and the environment are influenced by the patterns of space occupation. Therefore, the use of geoprocessing techniques to analyze the spatial distribution of health problems allows one to determine local risks and delimit areas that concentrate the most vulnerable situations (occurrence of disease, characteristics of the environment and habitat of the intermediate host / vector). It is also possible with the use of geographic information systems to plan, schedule, control, monitor, and evaluate the diseases in groups according to their risk of transmission [12].

The use of Geographic Information Systems (GIS) and statistical tools in health has been facilitated by access to epidemiological data bases, enabling the production of thematic maps that contribute to the formulation of hypotheses about the spatial distribution of diseases and their relation to the socioeconomic variables [13].

The use of GIS and Remote Sensing (RS) are powerful tools for working complex analysis of a large number of information and viewing the results of this analysis in graphical maps. Since the seventies, RS has been applied to social sciences and health [14]. There are numerous information collected by RS data, describing some biotic and abiotic factors [15]. Application of RS and GIS techniques for mapping the risk of parasitic diseases, including schistosomiasis, has been performed over the past 15 years [16].

The estimate of schistosomiasis prevalence using GIS was first used in the Philippines and the Caribbean by [17, 18]. In Brazil, the use of GIS in schistosomiasis was first used by [19] in the state of Bahia. The authors constructed maps with environmental characteristics (total precipitation for three consecutive months, the annual maximum and minimum temperature and diurnal temperature differences), prevalence of *S. mansoni* and distribution of snails to study the spatial and temporal dynamics of infection and identify the environmental factors that influence the distribution of schistosomiasis. The results indicated that the snail population density and duration of annual dry season are the most important determinants for the prevalence of schistosomiasis in the study areas.

Table 1 shows a brief history of the use of GIS techniques in the study of schistosomiasis in several countries.

The main objective of the present study is to establish a relationship between schistosomiasis positivity index and the environmental and socioeconomic variables, in the Minas Gerais State, Brazil, using multiple linear regressions at small communities and cities levels.

Vector	Species	Study Area	Satellite-sensor	Technical-variables	Reference
-	*Schistosoma spp*	Philippines, theCaribbean	Landsat (MSS)	climate	[17, 18]
Oncomelania spp	*Schistosoma spp*	China	NOAA (AVHRR), Lansdat (TM)	ecological zones	[20]
B. truncatus, B. alexandrina	*S. mansoni, S. haematobium*	Egypt	NOAA (AVHRR)	temperature, NDVI	[21]
Phlebotomus papatasi	*Schistosoma spp*	Southeast Asia	NOAA (AVHRR)	NDVI	[22]
B. straminea	*S.mansoni*	Brazil	-	spatial distribution	[23]
B. pfeifferi	*S.mansoni*	Kenya	-	linear regression, mapping techniques, cluster analysis	[24]
B. alexandrina	*S. mansoni, S. haematobium*	Egypt	NOAA (AVHRR), Lansdat (TM)	dT, NDVI, MDE	[25]
B. glabrata, B. straminea, B. tenagophila	*S.mansoni*	Brazil	-	temperature, precipitation, DEM, soil type, vegetation type	[19]
Oncomelania spp	*Schistosoma spp*	China	Landsat (TM)	classification, GIS	[26]
Bulinus spp, *Biomphalaria* sp	*S. mansoni, S. haematobium*	Tanzania	-	GIS, logistic regression	[27]
B. alexandrina	*S. mansoni*	Egypt	NOAA (AVHRR), Lansdat (TM)	dT, BED, NDVI	[28]
B. glabrata, B. straminea	*S. mansoni*	Brazil	NOAA (AVHRR)	NDVI, dT	[29]
Bulinus spp	*S. haematobium*	Tanzania	NOAA (AVHRR)	LST, NDVI, DEM, precipitation, logistic regression	[30]
B. pfeifferi	*S. mansoni*	Ethiopia	NOAA (AVHRR)	LST, NDVI	[31]
B. pfeifferi	*S. mansoni*	Ethiopia	NOAA (AVHRR)	NDVI, temperature, logistic regression	[32]
Oncomelania spp	*S. japonicum*	China	NOAA (AVHRR), Lansdat (TM)	TNDVI	[33]
-	*Schistosoma spp*	Chad, Cameroon	NOAA (AVHRR)	ecology	[34]

Vector	Species	Study Area	Satellite-sensor	Technical-variables	Reference
B. pfeifferi, B. senegalensis	*S. mansoni, S. haematobium*	Africa (sub-Saharan Africa)	NOAA (AVHRR)	SIG	[35]
-	*S. haematobium*	Chad	-	environmental data	[36]
-	*S. mansoni, S. haematobium*	Cameroon	NOAA (AVHRR), EROS	logistic regression	[37]
Oncomelania spp	*Schistosoma spp*	China	Landsat (TM)	RS	[38]
Oncomelania hupensis	*S. japonicum*	China	Landsat (TM)	LU	[39]
Oncomelania spp, *Bulinus* spp, *Biomphalaria* spp	*S. japonicum, S. mansoni, S. haematobium*	China	Landsat (TM)	SIG	[40]
Oncomelania hupensis	*S. japonicum*	China	Lansdat (TM)	TNDVI	[41]
Bulinus spp.	*S. haematobium*	Kenya	NOAA (AVHRR)	Tmax	[42]
B. glabrata	*S. mansoni*	Brazil	-	GPS	[43]
-	*S. mansoni, S. haematobium*	Uganda	Landsat (TM)	ecological zones	[44]
-	*Schistosoma spp*	Uganda	NOAA (AVHRR)	LST	[45]
Oncomelania hupensis	*S. japonicum*	Japan	-	PDA	[46]
Oncomelania hupensis	*S. japonicum*	China	Ikonos, ASTER	MDE	[47]
-	*S. mansoni*	Côte d'Ivoire	Landsat (ETM), NOAA (AVHRR), EROS, MODIS	environmental and socioeconomic data	[16, 48]
O. hupensis	*S. japonicum*	China	Landsat (TM)	NDVI	[49]
Oncomelania hupensis	*S. japonicum*	China	NOAA (AVHRR)	LST	[50]
Oncomelania hupensis	*S. japonicum*	China	Landsat (TM)	SAVI	[51]

Vector	Species	Study Area	Satellite-sensor	Technical-variables	Reference
-	*S. mansoni*	Brazil	-	logistic regression models and Bayesian spatial models	[52]
Biomphalaria sp	*S.mansoni*	Brazil	MODIS, SRTM	regression, elevation, mixture model, NDVI	[53]
B. glabrata	*S.mansoni*	Brazil	-	spatial analysis, GPS, immunological data	[54]
Biomphalaria sp	*S.mansoni*	Brazil	-	social and environmental data, regression	[55]
Biomphalaria spp	*S. mansoni*	Brazil	-	GPS and GIS	[56]
B. glabrata	*S. mansoni*	Brazil	-	kernel	[57]
-	*Schistosoma spp*	Africa	-	ecology, GIS, RS, geostatistics	[58]
B. pfeifferi	*S. mansoni*	Côte d'Ivoire	-	socioeconomic data, logistic regression, Bayesian model	[59]
B. sudanica, B. stanleyi	*S. mansoni*	Uganda	-	spatial analysis	[60]
-	*S. haematobium*	Tanzania	-	social and ecological data, Bayesian models, logistic regression, NDVI, elevation, cluster analysis	[61]
Biomphalaria sp	*S.mansoni*	Brazil	MODIS, SRTM	social and environmental data, RS, NDVI, temperature, regression	[62]
Biomphalaria sp	*S.mansoni*	Brazil	MODIS, SRTM	linear regression, imprecise classification, regionalization and pattern recognition	[63]
Oncomelania hupensis	*S. japonicum*	China	SPOT	ecological data, land use, land cover, classification, Bayesian model, RS, NDVI, slope, LST	[64]
-	*Schistosoma spp*	China	-	GIS, spatial analysis and clustering, Bayesian model,	[65]
-	*S. mansoni, S. haematobium*	Mali	NOAA (AVHRR)	Bayesian models, NDVI, LST, GIS, logistic regression	[66]
Biomphalaria sp	*S.mansoni*	Brazil	-	kriging, spatial distribution	[67, 68]
Biomphalaria sp	*S.mansoni*	Brazil	-	Fuzzy logic	[69]

Vector	Species	Study Area	Satellite-sensor	Technical-variables	Reference
-	*S. japonicum*	China	-	GIS, spatial analysis, clustering, kernel	[70]
Biomphalaria sp	*S. mansoni*	Brazil	MODIS	meteorological data, socioeconomic, sanitation, RS, regression	[71]
B. straminea	*S.mansoni*	Brazil	-	kernel, GPS, spatial distribution	[72]
B. glabrata	*S.mansoni*	Brazil	MODIS	mixture model	[73]
Biomphalaria sp	*S.mansoni*	Brazil	MODIS, SRTM	social and environmental data, sanitation, biological, RS, NDVI, temperature, regression, kriging	[1, 74]
Biomphalaria sp	*S.mansoni*	Brazil	MODIS	decision tree, environmental data, RS	[75]
-	*S. mansoni*, *S. haematobium*	East Africa	-	Bayesian geostatistics, logistic regression, Markov chain Monte Carlo simulation,	[76]
Biomphalaria sp	*S.mansoni*	Africa	MODIS	Climate change, spatial distribution, temperature, precipitation, MaxEnt, soil	[77]
-	*S.mansoni*	Ethiopia, Kenya	NOAA (AVHRR)	geostatistics, LST, NDVI, elevation, environmental data, LQAS, LpCP	[78]
Biomphalaria spp	*S. mansoni*	Brazil	-	GPS, GIS, spatial distribution	[79]

Table 1. Use of geoprocessing techniques in the study of schistosomiasis.

2. Material and methods

2.1. Materials

The study area includes 4,846 small communities (called localities) in the entire State of Minas Gerais, Brazil. The dependent variable is the schistosomiasis positivity index (*Ip*). *Ip* were obtained from the Brazilian Schistosomiasis Control Program (PCE) through the annual reports of the Secretary of Public Health Surveillance (SVS) and the Secretary of Health in the State of Minas Gerais (SESMG). From the 4,846 locations mentioned above, only 1,590 of them have information on the positivity of the disease. Since schistosomiasis is a disease characterized by environmental and social factors, environmental and socioeconomic variables were used as explanatory variables, as well as a variable containing information about presence of intermediate hosts. A brief description of these variables is given below.

2.2. Schistosomiasis positivity index

Schistosomiasis positivity index (*Ip*) values were obtained in 1,590 localities from the Brazilian Schistosomiasis Control Program (PCE) through the Annual Reports of the Secretary of Public Health Surveillance (SVS) and the Secretary of Health in the State of Minas Gerais (SESMG). The *Ip* data were obtained from the database SISPCE (Information System of the Brazilian Schistosomiasis Control Program) from 1996 to 2009. The Kato-Katz technique is the methodology used to determine positivity index, examining one slide per person.

These *Ip* were determined for each locality *i* by:

$$Ip = \frac{r_i}{n_i} * 100 \tag{1}$$

where: r_i is the number of infected people and n_i is the total population in locality *i*.

2.3. Intermediate hosts

Information about the existence of *Biomphalaria* snails were provided at a municipality basis by the Laboratory of Helminthiasis and Medical Malacology of the Rene Rachou Research Center (CPqRR/Fiocruz-MG).

The distribution of Biomphalaria snails used for this study was defined as: *B. glabrata, B. tenagophila, B. straminea, B. glabrata + B. tenagophila, B. glabrata + B. straminea, B. tenagophila + B. straminea, B. glabrata + B. tenagophila + B. straminea* and No *Biomphalaria*. The class "No *Biomphalaria*" includes information about the non-occurrence of *Biomphalaria* species or information about non-transmitter species in Brazil, such as *B. peregrina, B. schrammi, B. intermedia, B. occidentalis*, etc.

The spatial distribution of the schistosomiasis *Ip* and the *Biomphalaria* species data are presented in Fig. 1.

2.4. Environmental data

Twenty eight environmental variables were obtained from remote sensing and meteorological sources.

The remote sensing variables were derived from Moderate Resolution Imaging Spectroradiometer (MODIS) and from the Shuttle Radar Topography Mission (SRTM) sensor.

The variables of MODIS sensor used were collected in two seasons, summer (from 17/Jan/2002 to 01/Feb/2002 period) and winter (from 28/Jul/2002 to 12/Aug/2002 period). MODIS data were composed by the blue, red, near and middle infrared bands and also the vegetation indices (NDVI and EVI) [73].

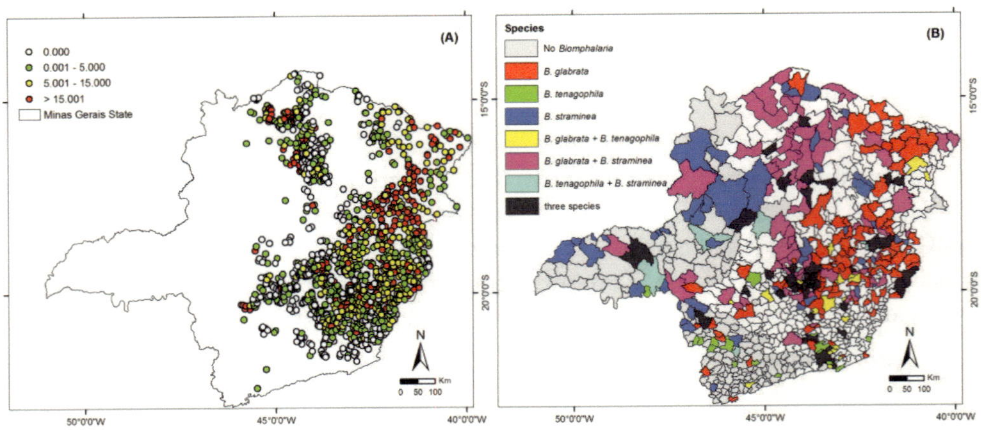

Figure 1. Spatial distribution of the (a) schistosomiasis and (b) *Biomphalaria* species in Minas Gerais State, Brazil.

The Linear Spectral Mixture Model (LSMM) is an image processing algorithm that generates fraction images with the proportion of each component (vegetation, soil, and shade) inside the pixel, which is estimated by minimizing the sum of square of the errors. In this work, the so called vegetation, soil, and shade fraction images were generated using the MODIS data, and the estimated values for the spectral reflectance components were also used as an input to the regression models [73].

Others variables obtained from SRTM were also used in this study: the digital elevation model (*DEM*) and slope (derived from *DEM*). Based on the SRTM data, a drainage map of Minas Gerais was generated, and the variables: water percentage in municipality (*QTA*) and water accumulation (*WA*) were derived. Six meteorological variables consisting of total precipitation (*Prec*), minimum (*Tmin*) and maximum (*Tmax*) temperature average for summer and winter seasons were obtained from the Center for Weather Forecast and Climate Studies (CPTEC), in the same date of MODIS images.

2.5. Socioeconomic data

Socioeconomic variables obtained by The Brazilian Institute of Geography and Statistics (IBGE) census for the year 2000 were also used as explanatory variables. The variables used in this work are those related to the water quality (percentage of domiciles with access to the general net of water supply, access to the water through wells or springheads, and with other access forms to the water), and to the sanitary conditions (the percentage of domiciles with bathroom connected to rivers or lakes, connected to a ditch, to rudimentary sewage, to septic sewage, to a general net, to other sewerage type, with bathroom or sanitarium and without bathroom or sanitarium).

2.6. Methods

Indicator kriging and multiple linear regressions were employed to estimate the presence of the intermediate host and the schistosomiasis disease, respectively.

2.7. Indicator Kriging

Since information about existence of *Biomphalaria* is only available on municipality basis, indicator kriging was used in this study to make inferences, in a grid basis, about the presence of the *Biomphalaria* species (*B. glabrata, B. tenagophila* and/or *B. straminea*), intermediate hosts of *S. mansoni*. The method allows spatialization of the data conditioned to the sample set of categorical attributes, aiming at the spatial distribution and production of maps.

The categorical attributes (classes) used for this study were defined as: *B. glabrata, B. tenagophila, B. straminea, B. glabrata* + *B. tenagophila, B. glabrata* + *B. straminea, B. tenagophila* + *B. straminea, B. glabrata* + *B. tenagophila* + *B. straminea* and No *Biomphalaria* totalizing eight probable classes.

The snail attributes (class of species and localization) were distributed along the drainage network of 15 River Basins (Buranhém, Doce, Grande, Itabapoana, Itanhém, Itapemirim, Jequitinhonha, Jucuruçu, Mucuri, Paraíba do Sul, Paranaíba, Pardo, Piracicaba/Jaguari, São Francisco and São Mateus), according to the methodology used by [67].

In [1], however the indicator kriging was used only at municipalities' level, but in this study it was used for localities level.

Indicator kriging procedures were applied to obtain an approximation of the conditional distribution function of the random variables. Based on the estimated function, maps of snail spatial distributions along with the corresponding uncertainties for the entire state and also map of estimated prevalence of schistosomiasis were built.

The indicator kriging result was used as a variable in multiple regression models.

2.8. Multiple linear regressions

Multiple linear regressions are a form of regression analysis in which data are modeled by a least squares function which is a linear combination of the model parameters and depends on one or more independent variables.

The regression analysis was applied with the schistosomiasis *Ip* as dependent variable, in addition to 93 quantitative variables (28 environmental variables and 65 socioeconomic variables), and one qualitative variable resulting from the kriging (presence or absence of *B. glabrata*) as explanatory variables.

The dependent variable was randomly divided into two sets: one with 852 cases (localities) for variables selection and model definition, and another with 738 cases for model validation.

Due to the high number of independent variables, some procedures were performed for variables selection. The relations among the dependent and the independent variables were analyzed in terms of correlation, multi co-linearity, and possible transformations that better explain the dependent variable.

A logarithmic transformation for the dependent variable (denoted by *lnIp*) was made as it improved the correlation with independent variables.

The analysis of the correlation matrix showed that some variables had non-significative correlations with *lnIp* at 95% confidence level, and also some variables were highly correlated among themselves, indicating that those variables could be excluded from future analysis.

Since multi co-linearity effects among the remaining independent variables were detected, variables selection techniques were used in order to choose a set of variables that better explain the dependent variable. Variable selection was performed by the R^2 criterion using all possible regressions [80].

This selection technique consists in the identification of a best subset with few variables and a coefficient of determination R^2 sufficiently close to that when all variables are used in the model.

Interaction effects were also analyzed to be included in the model. After performing the residual analysis, the chosen regression model was then validated. The final estimated regression function was computed using the entire data set (definition and validation), and it was applied to all localities to build a risk map for schistosomiasis positivity index.

The multiple regressions were developed based on two approaches: a global model (throughout the state) and a regional model (regionalization).

Regionalization is a classification procedure using the SKATER algorithm (Spatial 'K'luster Analysis by Tree Edge Removal) applied to spatial objects with an areal representation (municipalities), which groups them into homogeneous contiguous regions [81].

Regionalization was applied in Minas Gerais to divide the state into four homogeneous regions. The choice of the number of regions was based on the spatial distribution of localities (Figure 1b) in order to achieve an adequate number of localities in each region.

The regional model was developed by doing a regression model separately in each of the four regions formed by first applying the SKATER algorithm using environmental variables [74].

The models validation was performed using the Root Mean Square Error (RMSE) and the Mean Squared Prediction Error (MSPR), given by [80].

$$RMSE = \sqrt{\frac{\sum_{i=1}^{n} \left(Ip_i - \hat{I}p_i \right)^2}{n}} \tag{2}$$

where Ip_i and $\hat{I}p_i$ represent, respectively, the observed and predicted positivity index in the i-th observation and n is the number of observations of the data model definition ($i = 1, \ldots, n$).

The RMSE measures the variation of the observed values around the estimated values. Ideally, the values of RMSE are close to zero. The MSPR is computed the same way as the RMSE, but using validation samples.

The final models were applied in all 4,846 localities to estimate the positivity index.

2.9. Simple average interpolator

The simple average interpolator (SAI) algorithm of the software SPRING [82] was used to estimate the value of *Ip* at each point (*x,y*) of the grid. This estimative is based on the simple average of the variable values in the eight nearest neighbors of this point, according to equation (3).

$$f(x,y) = \frac{1}{8}\left(\sum_{i=1}^{8} \hat{I}p_i\right) \tag{3}$$

where $\hat{I}p_i$ is the estimated positivity index of the 8 neighbors of the point (*x,y*) and *f*(*x,y*) is the interpolation function.

The file generated by interpolation was a grid with spatial resolution of 1 km. The purpose of using this tool was to determine which of the mesoregions presented estimated values above 15% (class with high positivity index).

3. Results and discussion

The GeoSchisto Database (http://www.dpi.inpe.br/geoschisto/) was created containing all variables used in this study.

The indicator kriging result was a regular grid of 250 x 250 meters with the estimate of *Biomphalaria* species class for the entire Minas Gerais State. The indicator kriging result is presented in Fig. 2a. The variable *B. glabrata* used in regression models is presented in Fig. 2b.

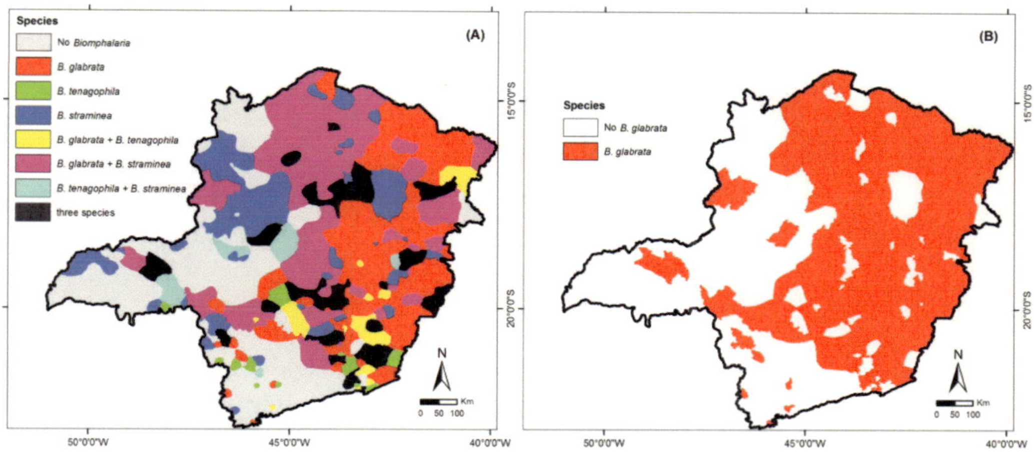

Figure 2. a) Kriging and (b) estimated presence of *B. glabrata* by indicator kriging.

3.1. Global model

The five variables selected were: presence or absence of the *B. glabrata*, summer precipitation (PC_s), summer minimum temperature (TN_s), winter Enhanced Vegetation Index (EVI_w) and households with a bathroom or toilet and sewage from septic tank type (V_{31}).

The final model, with $R^2 = 0.18$, was:

$$\widehat{Ip} = e^{(-7.34+0.51BG+0.004PC_s+0.37TN_s+0.0003EVI_w+0.004V_{31})} - 1 \quad (4)$$

Fig. 3a shows the estimated *Ip* for all 4,842 localities in Minas Gerais using the estimated regression equation (4). Figure 3b shows the plot of the residuals, resulting from the difference between observed and estimated *Ip* from 1,590 locations. In Figure 3b, dark colors (red and blue) represent overestimated values, light colors (red and blue) underestimated ones, and in white are the municipalities where the estimated prevalence differs very little from the true values.

The precipitation, minimum temperature, EVI and sanitation were positively correlated with *Ip*. This is consistent with the adequate environmental conditions for the transmission of schistosomiasis. Also, the transmission depends on the presence of *B. glabrata*.

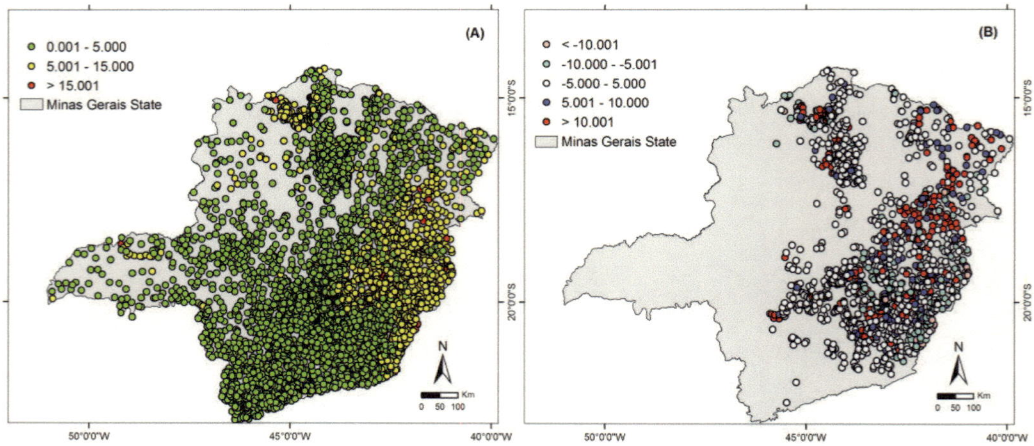

Figure 3. Global model: (a) estimated *Ip* and (b) residuals.

The result of this model has the same variables (*BG*, TN_s, Evi_w and sanitation) obtained by [74] when estimatives were done on a municipality basis, indicating a great similarity between the two global models. The difference is in the sanitation variable where the variable obtained by [74] was related to the type of water (well or spring) and this study to the type of sewage system (septic tank).

3.2. Regional model

The Minas Gerais State was divided into four regions using the SKATER algorithm. Table 2 presents the number of localities in each region used for model generation and for model validation. The regionalization can be seen in Figure 4 a.

	Model Generation	Model Validation	Total
Region 1 (R1)	104	66	170
Region 2 (R2)	428	262	690
Region 3 (R3)	220	338	558
Region 4 (R4)	100	72	172
Total	852	738	1590

Table 2. Number of localities in each region used for model generation and for model validation.

Regression models were developed for each of the four regions with the same 94 variables used in the global model, and the same selection procedure. Different numbers of variables were selected in each region to determine the best regression model.

The final models generated for each region (Fig. 4c) and their R^2 were:

$$\widehat{Ip}_1 = e^{(14.04+0.05PC_w+0.01V_{25}-1.15\Delta T_s)} - 1 \Rightarrow R^2 = 0.35 \tag{5}$$

$$\widehat{Ip}_2 = e^{(-11.63+0.68BG+0.59TN_s+0.0004EVI_w+0.03V_{25}-0.005V_{261})} - 1 \Rightarrow R^2 = 0.21 \tag{6}$$

$$\widehat{Ip}_3 = e^{(0.16+0.39BG+0.0002NDVI_s-0.015V_{33}+0.002V_{283})} - 1 \Rightarrow R^2 = 0.38 \tag{7}$$

$$\widehat{Ip}_4 = e^{(-3.54+0.0001EVI_s+0.006PC_s+0.16TN_s+0.27QTA+0.0006V_{254}+0.003V_{272})} - 1 \Rightarrow R^2 = 0.22 \tag{8}$$

where: PC_W (winter precipitation), V_{25} (percentage of households with another form of access to water), ΔT_S (difference of summer maximum and minimum temperature), BG (presence or not of the *B. glabrata*), TN_S (summer minimum temperature), EVI_W (winter Enhanced Vegetation Index), V_{261} (percentage of residents in households with another form of water supply), $NDVI_S$ (summer Normalized Difference Vegetation Index), V_{33} (percentage of housing with bathroom or toiled connected to a ditch), V_{283} (percentage of households without bathrooms), EVI_S (summer Enhanced Vegetation Index), PC_S (summer precipitation), QTA (water percentage in municipality), V_{254} (percentage of households with water supply network general) and V_{272} (percentage of households without toilet or sanitation).

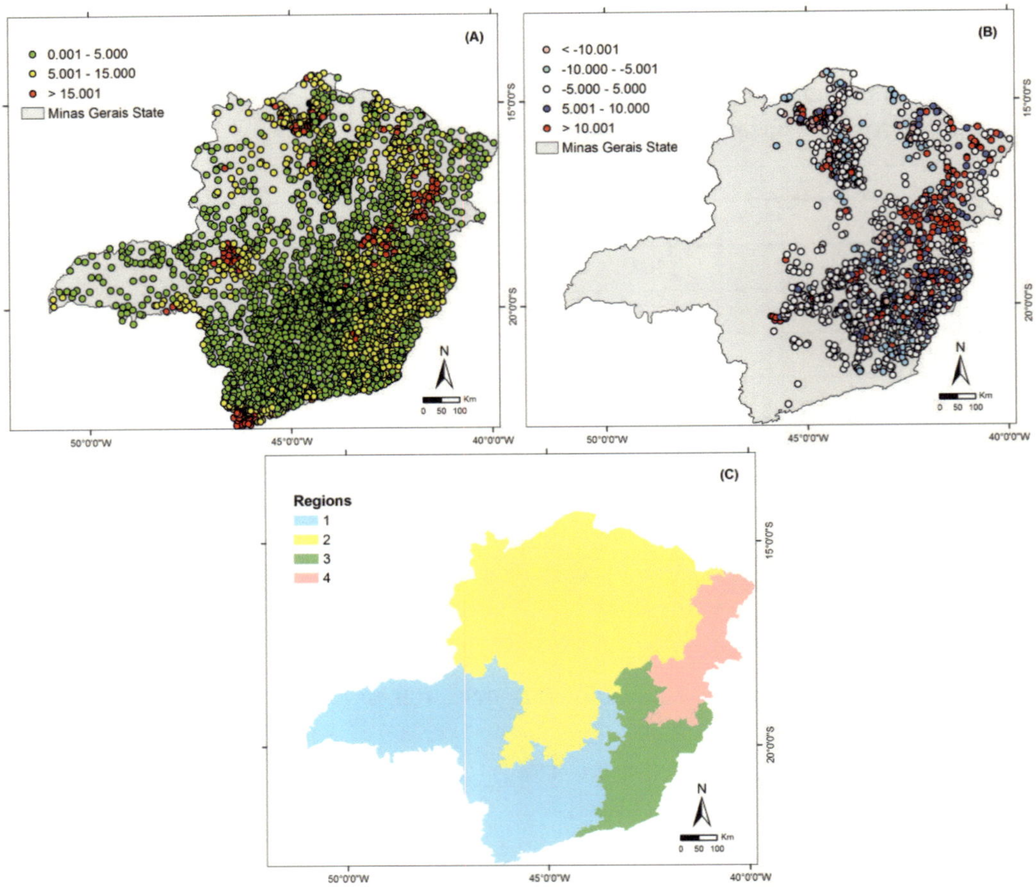

Figure 4. Regional model: (a) estimated *Ip*, (b) residuals. (c) regionalization.

Figure 4a shows the estimated values of *Ip* for all 4,842 localities in the Minas Gerais State using equations (3, 4, 5 and 6). Also, Figure 4b shows the residues from 1,590 locations. In this figure, red and blue represent overestimates, cyan and magenta represent the underestimated values and in the white localities with good estimate.

The regional model for Region 1 (R_1) reflects the effect of sanitation (households with other forms of water than tap water, wells or springs) and the influence of weather (precipitation and temperature of summer). Region 1 achieved a R^2 value of 0.35. The model obtained by [74] for the same Region 1 also has the same sanitation variable (percentage of homes with another type of access to water). The relationship between temperature and disease was also obtained by [29] and [55, 74].

The models for Regions 2 and 3 (R_2 and R_3) show the presence of *B. glabrata* associated with the effect of vegetation (Evi_w) and sanitation. Among the regional models, Region 2 had the lowest R^2 (0.21) and Region 3 had the highest R^2 (0.38).

The model for Region 4 (R_4) shows that *Ip* was associated with vegetation (Evi_s), weather (precipitation and temperature) and sanitation (type of water and sewage). The R^2 found for this model was 0.22.

In all models the presence of *B. glabrata,* sanitation, vegetation index and temperature were the most important variables. These characteristics are the same as environmental conditions for the presence and development of snails (infection of the intermediate host) and sanitation (water contamination - presence of *S. mansoni* cercariae) obtained by [74] which were obtained at municipalities level.

[29] also showed that the distribution of schistosomiasis in Bahia, at municipalities level, is related to the vegetation index (*NDVI*) and temperature (ΔTs) using sensor data from low spatial resolution (AVHRR/NOAA).

3.3. Simple Averages Interpolator (SAI)

Table 3 presents the mean square error (RMSE) and Mean Squared Error of Prediction (MSPR) for the global and regional models, for each region. From this table we can observe that the mean square decreased from 10.739 to 9.979 when we used separate models for each region. It was also noted that the RMSE of the Regional Model was smaller than the RMSE of the Global Model for all four regions, highlighting the importance of using different equations and different variables for each region. Since the Regional Model can be considered a better model the Simple Averages Interpolator (SAI), was applied using the known positivity index of the 1,590 localities (Fig. 5a), and using the regression estimated positivity index of all 4,842 localities (Fig. 5b). The objective of applying SAI to all estimated *Ip* values is to indicate current and potential local transmission of schistosomiasis.

	Model	n_{RMSE}	RMSE	n_{MSPR}	MSPR
Global	R_1	104	8.078	66	3.421
	R_2	428	12.369	262	11.741
	R_3	220	10.042	338	10.048
	R_4	100	6.164	72	8.282
	total	852	10.739	738	10.145
Regional	R_1	104	7.576	66	3.376
	R_2	428	11.553	262	11.577
	R_3	220	9.044	338	9.538
	R_4	100	6.123	72	8.291
	total	852	9.979	738	9.848

n (number of localities)

Table 3. Residual analysis of the dependent variable (*Ip*) for the models.

Figure 5a shows clusters presence in six mesoregions (Norte de Minas, Jequitinhonha, Vale do Mucuri, Vale do Rio Doce, Metropolitana de Belo Horizonte and Zona da Mata) with the highest *Ip* values. In Figure 5b the same six mesoregions can be noticed; however two news clusters in Sul/Sudoeste de Minas and Triângulo Mineiro/Alto Parnaíba mesoregions presented, respectively high and middle *Ip* values.

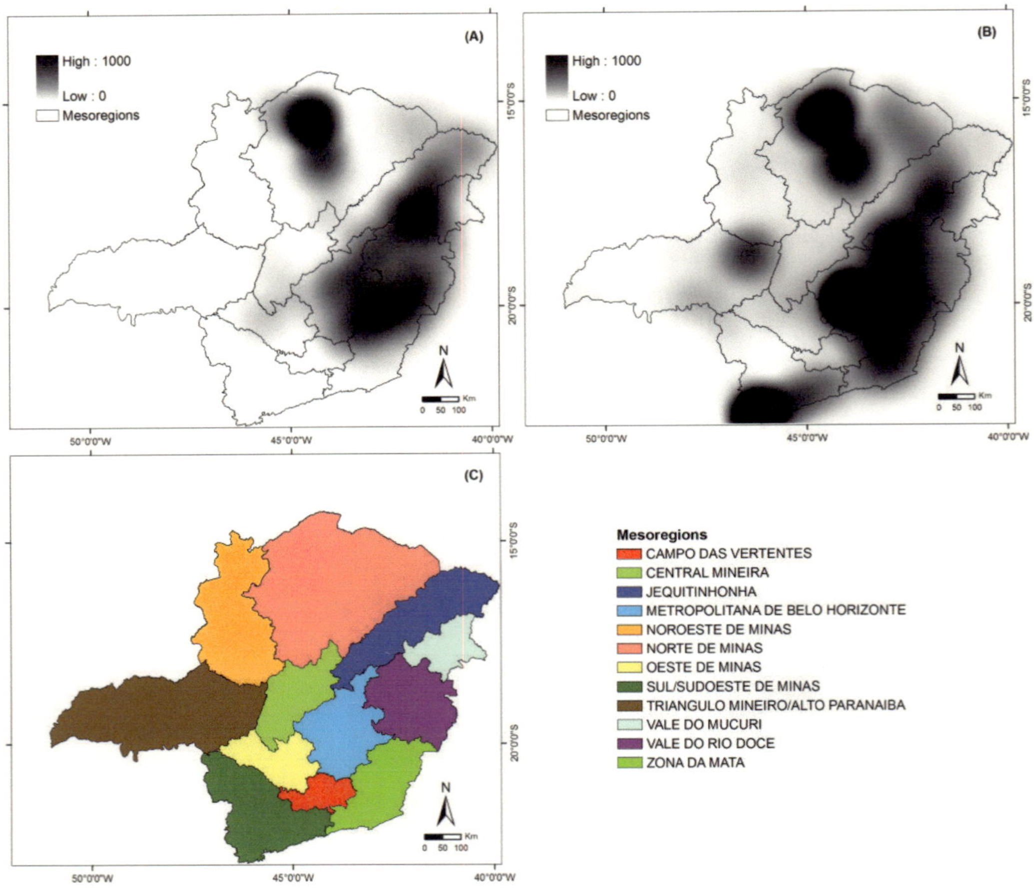

Figure 5. The averages interpolator: (a) *Ip* and (b) estimated *Ip* by Regional Model. (c) Mesoregions of Minas Gerais State.

Thus, the Norte de Minas, Jequitinhonha, Vale do Mucuri, Vale do Rio Doce, Metropolitana de Belo Horizonte and Zona da Mata mesoregions are endemics areas.

Sul/Sudoeste de Minas and Triângulo Mineiro/Alto Parnaíba mesoregions are not endemic areas, but have a schistosomiasis focus (Itajubá municipality in Sul mesoregion). The Sul/Sudoeste de Minas mesoregion has 146 municipalities representing about 20% of municipalities in Minas Gerais State and is a non-endemic area for schistosomiasis. Due to the high concentration of cities in an area of 49,523.893 km^2 (which represents less than 10% of the area of Minas Gerais State) and a high agricultural economy, it is a region with high risk of schistosomiasis transmission. Therefore, it would be interesting to do a detailed study in the Sul mesoregion to determine the schistosomiasis *Ip*.

Also, it would be interesting to keep surveillance in the municipalities of the Triângulo Mineiro/Alto Parnaíba mesoregion that presented *B. glabrata* presence.

4. Conclusions and future work

This study shows the importance of a joint use of GIS and RS to study the risk of schistosomiasis. Moreover, it can be concluded that the combined use of GIS and statistical techniques allowed the estimation of schistosomiasis *Ip*. Results of the regression models confirmed the importance of the use of environmental variables to characterize the snail habitat in the endemic area of the state of Minas Gerais.

Results of the regression models show that regionalization improves the estimation of the disease in Minas Gerais. Based on this model, a schistosomiasis risk map was built for Minas Gerais. [74] and [75] also obtained a better model with the use of regionalization when estimating schistosomiasis at a municipality level.

The Simple Averages Interpolator is a technique that may indicate possible local to transmission and surveillance of schistosomiasis.

It is recommended the use of GPS for field surveys together and the application of this methodology with images of better spatial resolution (10-30m) in other states for validation. Also, we recommend using a smaller area (municipality or mesoregion) estimate for the schistosomiasis.

The methodology used in this study can be utilized to control schistosomiasis in the areas with occurrence of the disease and also it can be used to take preventive measures to prevent the disease transmission.

Next step will be to utilize data from the PCE by localities to study other diseases such as ascariasis, hookworm, trichuriasis, etc, using data from CBERS and/or Landsat and new methodologies (Geographically Weighted Regression, Generalized Additive Model, etc).

Acknowledgements

The authors woud like to acknowledge the support of Sandra da Costa Drummond (Fundação Nacional de Saúde) and the support of CNPq (Conselho Nacional de Desenvolvimento Científico e Tecnológico) (grants # 300679/2011-4, 384571/2010-7, 302966/2009-9, 308253/2008-6).

Author details

Ricardo J.P.S. Guimarães[1*], Corina C. Freitas[2], Luciano V. Dutra[2], Guilherme Oliveira[3] and Omar S. Carvalho[3]

*Address all correspondence to: ricardojpsg@gmail.com

1 Instituto Evandro Chagas/IEC, Ananindeua, Brazil

2 Instituto Nacional de Pesquisas Espaciais/INPE, São José dos Campos, Brazil

3 Centro de Pesquisas René Rachou/Fiocruz-MG, Belo Horizonte, Brazil

References

[1] Guimarães RJPS, Fonseca FR, Dutra LV, Freitas CC, Oliveira GC, Carvalho OS. A study of schistosomiasis prevalence and risk of snails presence spatial distributions using geo-statistical tools. In: MB R, (ed.). Schistosomiasis. Rijeka: InTech, 2012. p255-80.

[2] Correa LR, Paraense WL. Susceptibility of *Biomphalaria amazonica* to infection with two strains of *Schistosoma mansoni*. Rev Inst Med Trop São Paulo. 1971;13 387-90.

[3] Paraense WL, Correa LR. Susceptibility of *Biomphalaria peregrina* from Brazil and Ecuador to two strains of *Schistosoma mansoni*. Rev Inst Med Trop São Paulo. 1973;15 127-30.

[4] Caldeira RL, Teodoro TM, Gomes MFB, Carvalho OS. Preliminary studies investigating the occurrence of *Biomphalaria cousini* in Brazil. Mem Inst Oswaldo Cruz. 2010;105(4) 485-7.

[5] Carvalho OS, Rocha RS, Massara CL, Katz N. Expansão da esquistossomose mansoni em Minas Gerais. Mem Inst Oswaldo Cruz. 1987;82(Suppl. IV) 295-8.

[6] Carvalho OS, Massara CL, Rocha RS, Katz N. Esquistossomose Mansoni no Sudoeste do Estado de Minas Gerais (Brasil). Rev Saúde Pública. 1989;23 341-4.

[7] Carvalho OS, Massara CL, Silveira Neto HV, Guerra HL, Caldeira RL, Mendonça CLF, et al. Re-evaluation of Schistosomiasis Mansoni in Minas Gerais, Brazil. II. Alto Paranaiba Mesoregion. Mem Inst Oswaldo Cruz. 1997;92 141-2.

[8] WHO. Study Group on the Ecology of Intermediate Snail Hosts of Bilharziasis. Geneva: World Health Organization; 1957.

[9] Juberg P, Schall VT, Barbosa JV, Gatti MJ, Soares MS. Behavior of *Biomphalaria glabrata*, the intermediate host snail of *Schistosoma mansoni*, at different depths in water in laboratory conditions. Mem Inst Oswaldo Cruz. 1987;82 179-208.

[10] Katz N, Carvalho OS. Introdução recente da esquistossomose mansoni no sul do estado de Minas Gerais, Brasil. Mem Inst Oswaldo Cruz. 1983;78 281-4.

[11] Carvalho OS, Rocha RS, Massara CL, Katz N. Primeiros casos autóctones de esquistossomose mansonica em região do noroeste do Estado de Minas Gerais (Brasil). Rev Saúde Pública São Paulo. 1988;22 237-9.

[12] Carvalho MS, Pina MF, Santos SM. Conceitos Básicos de Sistemas de Informação Geográfica e Cartografia Aplicados à Saúde. Brasília: OPS/Ministério da Saúde, 2000.

[13] Rojas LI, Barcellos C, Petter P. Utilização de mapas no campo da epidemiologia no Brasil. Informe Epidemiológico do SUS. 1999;8 25-35.

[14] Cline BL. New eyes for epidemiologists: aerial photography and other remote sensing techniques. Am J Epidemiol. 1970;92 85-9.

[15] Beck LR, Lobitz BM, Wood BL. Remote Sensing and Human Health: New Sensors and New Opportunities. Emerg Infect Dis. 2000;6(3) 217-27.

[16] Raso G, Matthys B, N'Goran EK, Tanner M, Vounatsou P, Utzinger J. Spatial risk prediction and mapping of *Schistosoma mansoni* infections among schoolchildren living in western Côte d'Ivoire. Parasitology. 2005;131(01) 97-108.

[17] Cross ER, Bailey RC. Prediction of areas endemic for schistosomiasis through use of discriminant analysis of environmental data. Mil Med. 1984;149 28-30.

[18] Cross ER, Sheffield C, Perrine R, Pazzaglia G. Predicting areas endemic for schistosomiasis using weather variables and a Landsat data base. Mil Med. 1984 Oct;149(10) 542-4.

[19] Bavia ME, Hale L, Malone JB, Braud DH, Shane SM. Geographic information systems and the enviromental risk of Schistosomiasis in Bahia, Brazil. Am J Trop Med Hyg. 1999;60(4) 566-72.

[20] Chen S, Hu J. Geo-ecological zones and endemic diseases in China -- a sample study by remote sensing. Preventive Veterinary Medicine. 1991;11(3-4) 335-44.

[21] Malone JB, Huh OK, Fehler DP, Wilson PA, Wilensky DE, Holmes RA, et al. Temperature data from satellite imagery and distribution of schistosomiasis in Egypt. Am J Trop Med Hyg. 1994;51(3) 714-22.

[22] Cross ER, Newcomb WW, Tucker CJ. Use of weather data and remote sensing to predict the geographic and seasonal distribution of *Phlebotomus papatasi* in southwest Asia. Am J Trop Med Hyg. 1996;54(5) 530-6.

[23] Teles HMS. Distribuição de *Biomphalaria straminea* ao Sul da Região Neotropical, Brasil. Rev Saude Publica. 1996;30(4) 341-9.

[24] Kloos H, Fulford AJC, Butterworth AE, Sturrock RF, Ouma JH, Kariuki HC, et al. Spatial patterns of human water contact and *Schistosoma mansoni* transmission and infection in four rural areas in Machakos District, Kenya. Social Science & Medicine. 1997;44(7) 949-68.

[25] Malone JB, Abdel-Rahman MS, El Bahy MM, Huh OK, Shafik M, Bavia M. Geographic information systems and the distribution of *Schistosoma mansoni* in the Nile delta. Parasitol Today. 1997;13(3) 112-9.

[26] Gong P, Spear R, Seto E, Zhou Y, Xu B, Maxzle D, et al. Remote sensing and GIS for schistosomiasis control in Sichuan, China, an overview. Proceedings of Geoinformatics'99; 1999 19-21 JUNE; Ann Arbor, MI; 1999. p. 1-9.

[27] Lwambo NJS, Siza JE, Brooker S, Bundy DAP, Guyatt H. Patterns of concurrent hookworm infection and schistosomiasis in schoolchildren in Tanzania. Transactions of the Royal Society of Tropical Medicine and Hygiene. 1999;93(5) 497-502.

[28] Abdel-Rahman MS, El-Bahy MM, Malone JB, Thompson RA, El Bahy NM. Geographic information systems as a tool for control program management for schistosomiasis in Egypt. Acta Trop. 2001;79(1) 49-57.

[29] Bavia ME, Malone JB, Hale L, Dantas A, Marroni L, Reis R. Use of thermal and vegetation index data from earth observing satellites to evaluate the risk of schistosomiasis in Bahia, Brazil. Acta Trop. 2001;79(1) 79-85.

[30] Brooker S, Hay SI, Issae W, Hall A, Kihamia CM, Lwambo NJ, et al. Predicting the distribution of urinary schistosomiasis in Tanzania using satellite sensor data. Trop Med Int Health. 2001 Dec;6(12) 998-1007.

[31] Kristensen TK, Malone JB, McCarroll JC. Use of satellite remote sensing and geographic information systems to model the distribution and abundance of snail intermediate hosts in Africa: a preliminary model for *Biomphalaria pfeifferi* in Ethiopia. Acta Trop. 2001;79(1) 73-8.

[32] Malone JB, Yilma JM, McCarroll JC, Erko B, Mukaratirwa S, Zhou X. Satellite climatology and the environmental risk of *Schistosoma mansoni* in Ethiopia and east Africa. Acta Trop. 2001;79(1) 59-72.

[33] Zhou XN, Malone JB, Kristensen TK, Bergquist NR. Application of geographic information systems and remote sensing to schistosomiasis control in China. Acta Trop. 2001;79(1) 97-106.

[34] Beasley M, Brooker S, Ndinaromtan M, Madjiouroum EM, Baboguel M, Djenguinabe E, et al. First nationwide survey of th health of schoolchildren in Chad. Trop Med Int Health. 2002;7(7) 625-30.

[35] Brooker S. Schistosomes, snails and satellites. Acta Tropica. 2002;82(2) 207-14.

[36] Brooker S, Beasley M, Ndinaromtan M, Madjiouroum EM, Baboguel M, Djenguinabe E, et al. Use of remote sensing and a geographic information system in a national helminth control programme in Chad. Bull World Health Organ. 2002;80 783-9.

[37] Brooker S, Hay SI, Tchuem Tchuenté LA, Ratard R. Using NOAA AVHRR data to model human helminth distribuitions in planning disease control in Cameroon. Photogrametric Engineering & Remote Sensing. 2002;68(2) 175-9.

[38] Davis GM, Wu WP, Chen HG, Liu HY, Guo J-G, Lin D-D, et al. A baseline study of importance of bovines for human *Schistosoma japonicum* infections around Poyang Lake, China: villages studied and snail sampling strategy. Am J Trop Med Hyg. 2002;66 359-71.

[39] Seto E, Xu B, Liang S, Gong P, Wu W, Davis GM, et al. The use of remote sensing for predictive modeling of schistosomiasis in China. Photogramm Eng Rem Sens. 2002;68(2) 167-74.

[40] Zhou X, Acosta L, Willingham AL, Leonardo LR, Minggang C, Aligui G, et al. Regional Network for Research, Surveillance and Control of Asian Schistosomiasis (RNAS). Acta Trop. 2002;82(2) 305-11.

[41] Zhou X, Dandan L, Huiming Y, Honggen C, Leping S, Guojing Y, et al. Use of landsat TM satellite surveillance data to measure the impact of the 1998 flood on snail intermediate host dispersal in the lower Yangtze River Basin. Acta Trop. 2002;82(2) 199-205.

[42] McNally K. Developing Risk Assessment Maps For *Schistosoma Haematobium* Based On Climate Grids And Remotely Sensed Data: Louisiana State University; 2003.

[43] Barbosa CS, Araújo KC, Antunes L, Favre T, Pieri OS. Spatial distribution of schistosomiasis foci on Itamaracá Island, Pernambuco, Brazil. Mem Inst Oswaldo Cruz. 2004;99(Suppl. I) 79-83.

[44] Brooker S, Kabatereine NB, Clements ACA, Stothard JR. Schistosomiasis control. The Lancet. 2004;363 658-9.

[45] Kabatereine NB, Brooker S, Tukahebwa EM, Kazibwe F, Onapa AW. Epidemiology and geography of *Schistosoma mansoni* in Uganda: implications for planning control. Trop Med Int Health. 2004;9(3) 372-80.

[46] Nihei N, Kajihara N, Kirinoki M, Chigusa Y, Saitoh Y, Shimamura R, et al. Fixed-point observation of *Oncomelania nosophora* in Kofu Basin--establishment of monitoring system of schistosomiasis japonica in Japan. Parasitology International. 2004;53 199-205.

[47] Xu B, Gong P, Biging G, Liang S, Seto E, Spear R. Snail Density Prediction for Schistosomiasis Control Using Ikonos and ASTER Images. Photogram Eng Rem S. 2004;70(11) 1285-94.

[48] Raso G, Vounatsou P, Singer BH, N'Goran EK, Tanner M, Utzinger J. An integrated approach for risk profiling and spatial prediction of *Schistosoma mansoni* – hookworm coinfection. PNAS. 2006;103(18) 6934-9.

[49] Guo J-G, Penelope V, Cao C-L, Jurg U, Zhu H-Q, Daniel A, et al. A geographic information and remote sensing based model for prediction of *Oncomelania hupensis* habitats in the Poyang Lake area, China. Acta Tropica. 2005;96(2-3) 213-22.

[50] Yang G-J, Vounatsou P, Zhou X-N, Tanner M, Utzinger J. A Bayesian-based approach for spatio-temporal modeling of county level prevalence of *Schistosoma japoni-*

cum infection in Jiangsu province, China. International Journal for Parasitology. 2005;35(2) 155-62.

[51] Zhang Z-Y, Xu D-Z, Zhou X-N, Zhou Y, Liu S-J. Remote sensing and spatial statistical analysis to predict the distribution of *Oncomelania hupensis* in the marshlands of China. Acta Trop. 2005;96(2-3) 205-12.

[52] Brooker S, Alexander N, Geiger S, Moyeed RA, Stander J, Fleming F, et al. Contrasting patterns in the small-scale heterogeneity of human helminth infections in urban and rural environments in Brazil. International Journal for Parasitology. 2006;36(10-11) 1143-51.

[53] Freitas CC, Guimarães RJPS, Dutra LV, Martins FT, Gouvea EJC, Santos RAT, et al. Remote Sensing and Geographic Information Systems for the Study of Schistosomiasis in the State of Minas Gerais, Brazil. Geoscience and Remote Sensing Symposium, 2006 IGARSS 2006 IEEE International Conference on; 2006 July 31 2006-Aug. 4 2006; 2006. p. 2436-9.

[54] Gazzinelli A, LoVerde PT, Haddad JPA, Pereira WR, Bethony J, Correa-Oliveira R, et al. The spatial distribution of *Schistosoma mansoni* infection before and after chemotherapy in the Jequitinhonha Valley in Brazil. Mem Inst Oswaldo Cruz. 2006;101(Suppl. I) 63-71.

[55] Guimarães RJPS, Freitas CC, Dutra LV, Moura ACM, Amaral RS, Drummond SC, et al. Analysis and estimative of schistosomiasis prevalence for Minas Gerais state, Brazil, using multiple regression with social and environmental spatial data. Mem Inst Oswaldo Cruz. 2006;101(Suppl. I) 91-6.

[56] Tibiriçá SHC. Identificação morfológica e molecular, biometria, abundância e distribuição geográfica de *Biomphalaria* spp (Preston, 1910) (Mollusca, Planorbidae) no município de Juiz de Fora, Minas Gerais. MSc thesis.Universidade Federal de Juiz de Fora; 2006.

[57] Araújo KCGM, Resendes APC, Souza-Santos R, Silveira Júnior JC, Barbosa CS. Análise espacial dos focos de *Biomphalaria glabrata* e de casos humanos de esquistossomose mansônica em Porto de Galinhas, Pernambuco, Brasil, no ano 2000. Cadernos de Saúde Pública. 2007;23 409-17.

[58] Brooker S. Spatial epidemiology of human schistosomiasis in Africa: risk models, transmission dynamics and control. Trans R Soc Trop Med Hyg. 2007;101(1) 1-8.

[59] Matthys B, Tschannen AB, Tian-Bi NT, Comoé H, Diabaté S, Traoré M, et al. Risk factors for *Schistosoma mansoni* and hookworm in urban farming communities in western Côte d'Ivoire. Tropical Medicine & International Health. 2007;12(6) 709-23.

[60] Moira AP, Fulford AJC, Kabatereine NB, Kazibwe F, Ouma JH, Dunne DW, et al. Microgeographical and tribal variations in water contact and *Schistosoma mansoni* exposure within a Ugandan fishing community. Tropical Medicine & International Health. 2007;12(6) 724-35.

[61] Clements ACA, Brooker S, Nyandindi U, Fenwick A, Blair L. Bayesian spatial analysis of a national urinary schistosomiasis questionnaire to assist geographic targeting of schistosomiasis control in Tanzania, East Africa. International Journal for Parasitology. 2008;38(3-4) 401-15.

[62] Guimarães RJPS, Freitas CC, Dutra LV, Moura ACM, Amaral RS, Drummond SC, et al. Schistosomiasis Risk Estimation in Minas Gerais State, Brazil, using Environmental Data and GIS techniques. Acta Trop. 2008;108 234-41.

[63] Martins FT. Mapeamento do risco da esquistossomose no estado de Minas Gerais, usando dados ambientais e sociais. MSc thesis. INPE; 2008.

[64] Yang K, Wang X-H, Yang G-J, Wu X-H, Qi Y-L, Li H-J, et al. An integrated approach to identify distribution of *Oncomelania hupensis*, the intermediate host of *Schistosoma japonicum*, in a mountainous region in China. International Journal for Parasitology. 2008;38(8-9) 1007-16.

[65] Zhang Z, Carpenter TE, Chen Y, Clark AB, Lynn HS, Peng W, et al. Identifying high-risk regions for schistosomiasis in Guichi, China: A spatial analysis. Acta Trop. 2008;107 217-23.

[66] Clements ACA, Bosqué-Oliva E, Sacko M, Landouré A, Dembélé R, Traoré M, et al. A Comparative Study of the Spatial Distribution of Schistosomiasis in Mali in 1984-1989 and 2004-2006. PLoS Negl Trop Dis. 2009;3(5) e431.

[67] Guimarães RJPS, Freitas CC, Dutra LV, Felgueiras CA, Moura ACM, Amaral RS, et al. Spatial distribution of *Biomphalaria* mollusks at São Francisco River Basin, Minas Gerais, Brazil, using geostatistical procedures. Acta Trop. 2009;109 181-6.

[68] Guimarães RJPS, Freitas CC, Dutra LV, Felgueiras CA, Drummond SC, Oliveira G, et al. Use of Indicator Kriging to Investigate Schistosomiasis in Minas Gerais State, Brazil. J Trop Med. 2012;2012(Article ID 837428) 10.

[69] Martins-Bedé FT, Godo L, Sandri S, Dutra LV, Freitas CC, Carvalho OS, et al. Classification of Schistosomiasis Prevalence Using Fuzzy Case-Based Reasoning. Bio-Inspired Systems: Computational and Ambient Intelligence: Berlin/Heidelberg, 2009. p8.

[70] Zhang Z, Clark AB, Bivand R, Chen Y, Carpenter TE, Peng W, et al. Nonparametric spatial analysis to detect high-risk regions for schistosomiasis in Guichi, China. Transactions of the Royal Society of Tropical Medicine and Hygiene. 2009;103(10) 1045-52.

[71] Carvalho OS, Scholte RGC, Guimarães RJPS, Freitas CC, Drummond SC, Amaral RS, et al. The Estrada Real project and endemic diseases: the case of schistosomiasis, geoprocessing and tourism. Mem Inst Oswaldo Cruz. 2010;105(4) 532-6.

[72] Galvão AF, Favre TC, Guimarães RJPS, Pereira APB, Zani LC, Felipe KT, et al. Spatial distribution of *Schistosoma mansoni* infection before and after chemotherapy with two praziquantel doses in a community of Pernambuco, Brazil. Mem Inst Oswaldo Cruz. 2010;105(4) 555-62.

[73] Guimarães RJPS, Freitas CC, Dutra LV, Scholte RGC, Amaral RS, Drummond SC, et al. Evaluation of a linear spectral mixture model and vegetation indices (NDVI and EVI) in a study of schistosomiasis mansoni and *Biomphalaria glabrata* distribution in the state of Minas Gerais, Brazil. Mem Inst Oswaldo Cruz. 2010;105(4) 512-8.

[74] Guimarães RJPS, Freitas CC, Dutra LV, Scholte RGC, Martins-Bedé FT, Fonseca FR, et al. A geoprocessing approach for studying and controlling schistosomiasis in the state of Minas Gerais, Brazil. Mem Inst Oswaldo Cruz. 2010;105(4) 524-31.

[75] Martins-Bedé FT, Dutra LV, Freitas CC, Guimarães RJPS, Amaral RS, Drummond SC, et al. Schistosomiasis risk mapping in the state of Minas Gerais, Brazil, using a decision tree approach, remote sensing data and sociological indicators. Mem Inst Oswaldo Cruz. 2010;105(4) 541-8.

[76] Schur N, HürSchur N, Stensgaard A, Chimfwembe K, Mushinge G, Simoonga C, et al. Spatially explicit Schistosoma infection risk in eastern Africa using Bayesian geostatistical modeling. Acta Trop. 2011. In Press. http://dx.doi.org/10.1016/j.actatropica.2011.10.006

[77] Stensgaard A-S, Utzinger J, Vounatsou P, Hürlimann E, Schur N, Saarnak CFL, et al. Large-scale determinants of intestinal schistosomiasis and intermediate host snail distribution across Africa: Does climate matter? Acta Trop. 2011. In Press. http://dx.doi.org/10.1016/j.actatropica.2011.11.010

[78] Sturrock HJW, Gething PW, Ashton RA, Kolaczinski JH, Kabatereine NB, Brooker S. Planning schistosomiasis control: investigation of alternative sampling strategies for *Schistosoma mansoni* to target mass drug administration of praziquantel in East Africa. International Health.3(3) 165-75.

[79] Tibiriça SHC, Mittherofhe A, Castro MF, Lima AC, Gonçalves M, Pinheiro IO, et al. Malacological survey of *Biomphalaria* snails in municipalities along the *Estrada Real* in the southeast of the State of Minas Gerais, Brazil. Rev Soc Bras Med Trop. 2011;44(2) 163-7.

[80] Neter J, Kutner MH, Nachtssheim CJ, Wasserman W. Applied linear statistical models. Boston: WCB/McGraw-Hill, 1996.

[81] Assunção RM, Neves MC, Camara G, Freitas CC. Efficient regionalization techniques for socio-economic geographical units using minimum spanning trees. Int J Geogr Inf Sci. 2006;20 797-811.

[82] INPE. SPRING V.4.1 Sistema de Processamento de Informações Georeferenciadas http://www.dpi.inpe.br/spring/. 2005.

Chapter 2

Epidemiological Survey of Human and Veterinary Schistosomiasis

I.S. Akande and A.A. Odetola

Additional information is available at the end of the chapter

http://dx.doi.org/10.5772/53523

1. Introduction

1.1. Incidence of schistosomiasis

Schistosomiasis is one of the fifteen neglected tropical diseases (NTDS) namely: schistosomiasis, ascariasis, buruli ulcer, chagas disease, cysticercosis, food borne trematodiases, hookworm disease, leprosy,lymphatic filariasis, trachoma, trichuriasis, leishmaniasis, guinea worm, trypanosomiasis and oncocerciasis. It is a resurgent disease and *Schistosoma* sp. Infects well over 250 million people worldwide beside livestock [1]. Schistosomiasis (also called Bilharzias after the German tropical disease specialist, Theodore M. Bilharz, 1829 – 1862) is second only to malaria in parasitic disease morbidity. Despite control programmes in place, the distribution and the number of people estimated to be infected or at risks have not reduced. Approximately, over 600 million people in tropical and subtropical countries are at risk and of those infected120 million are symptomatic with 20 million having severe manifestations. Schistosomiasis is endemic in many countries, not only in sub-Saharan Africa, but the Middle East, Far East, South and Central America and the Caribbean. It is endemic in about 76 countries of the world including Nigeria. Presently, an estimated 3 million Nigerian children aged between 5 and 14 years are infected.

Endemic distribution: Ten species of schistosomes can infect humans out of seventeen recognized species, but a vast majority of infections are caused by *Schistosomamansoni*, S. *japonicum* and S. *haematobium*. Today, 85% of the numbers of infected people live in sub-Saharan Africa due to ignorance, cultural beliefs and practices and water contact patterns where S. *mansoni*, S. *haematobium* and S *intercalatum* are endemic. Livestock such as cattle harbour *Schistosoma* bovis; sheep harbour *Schistosoma curassoni* among others. The crucial agent perpetuating this disease is the water based snail intermediate host, flourishing in slow moving waters of man-made lakes, dams, irrigations channels and other fresh water bodies important for increasing agricultural production in developing countries.

In Nigeria, *Bulinus globosus* (Morelet) and *Bulinus rohlfsi* (Clessin) are intermediate hosts of S. *haematobium* and they are widely distributed.

Symptoms: In the early stages of infection, symptoms include cough, headache, loss of appetite, aches and pains, and difficulty in breathing usually followed initial skin irritation. Nausea is common in more advanced infection, accompanied by haematuria and in some cases renal obstruction. *S. haematobium* infections usually come with haematuria, leukocyturia, urinary tract complaints, tender abdomen and supra-pubic tenderness whose outcome include chronic iron deficiency anaemia, scarring, deformity of the ureters and bladder, and chronic bacterial super infection. These could lead to severe damage of urinary tract organs, and ultimately to renal failure. Schistosomiasis generally is insidious, it begins harmlessly but the end can be fatal if no attention is given to it at the onset.

Medical treatment: Current medical management of bilharziasis relies on praziquantel, sometimes in combination with oxamniquine. Praziquantel (Biltriciide®, Bayer AG, Germany) a heterocyclic prazino-isoquinoline, is highly effective against all species of schistosomes pathogenic to humans. However, since its first use, praziquantel treatment has been noted not to be 100% effective in eliminating *S. haematobium* infection. In adult schistosomes, praziquantel reduces vesication, vacuolization, and disintegration of the tegument. It also causes mature schistosome eggs to hatch. Immature eggs remain unaffected and continue to develop to maturity. In longitudinal studies, bladder wall pathology and hydronephrosis have been found to regress upon treatment, especially in active phases of the infection. However, if chronic stricture of the ureters has occurred, no significant reduction of the renal collecting system may result. In such a case, surgical intervention including mechanical dilation, resection, re-implantation, formation of an ileal ureter, and even nephro-ureterectomy may be required.

Another concern with respect to the future of praziquantel treatment is the ever-present worry over the emergence of drug resistance. Praziquantel has been in use for 4 decades, during which time it has been the drug of choice for many human and veterinary parasitic infections worldwide. The European Commission has established an International Initiative of Praziquantel Use to review reports of low efficacy in clinical trials in Senegal and Egypt, and reports of resistant *S. mansoni* strain isolated in the laboratory. While investigations suggest that no emergence of praziquantel resistance in *S. haematobium* has yet occurred, mathematical models predict that such resistance can be expected to occur as early as 2010. As a consequence new drug is being actively investigated.

Vaccines: No effective vaccine is yet available against any of the *Schistosoma* species. The Schistosoma Genome Project, created in 1992, has begun to yield comprehensive understanding of the molecular mechanism involved in schistosome nutrition and metabolism, host-dependent development and maturation, immune evasion, and invertebrate evolution. New potential vaccine candidates and drug targets are emerging.

The Life Cycle and Pathophysiology of *S. haematobium:* When eggs are excreted into fresh water, they hatch to release motile, ciliated miracidia (embryos) that penetrate aquatic bulinid snails, the intermediate host (Figures 1-3). Cercariae (larvae) emerges from the snails and penetrates the skin of humans in contact with the water (Figure 1). The cercaria (now called schistosomu-

http://dx.doi.org/10.5772/53523

lum) migrates to the lungs and liver, and after 6 weeks, the mature worms mate and migrate into the pelvic veins to begin oviposition. The eggs penetrate small, thin-walled vessels in the genitourinary system. During the active phase, viable adult worms deposit eggs that induce a granulomatous response with the formation of polyploidy lesions. During this phase eggs are excreted. An inactive phase follows the death of adult worms. No viable eggs are present in the urine and large numbers of calcified eggs are present in the wall of the bladder and other affected tissues. As fibrosis progresses, polypoid patches flatten into finely granular patches.

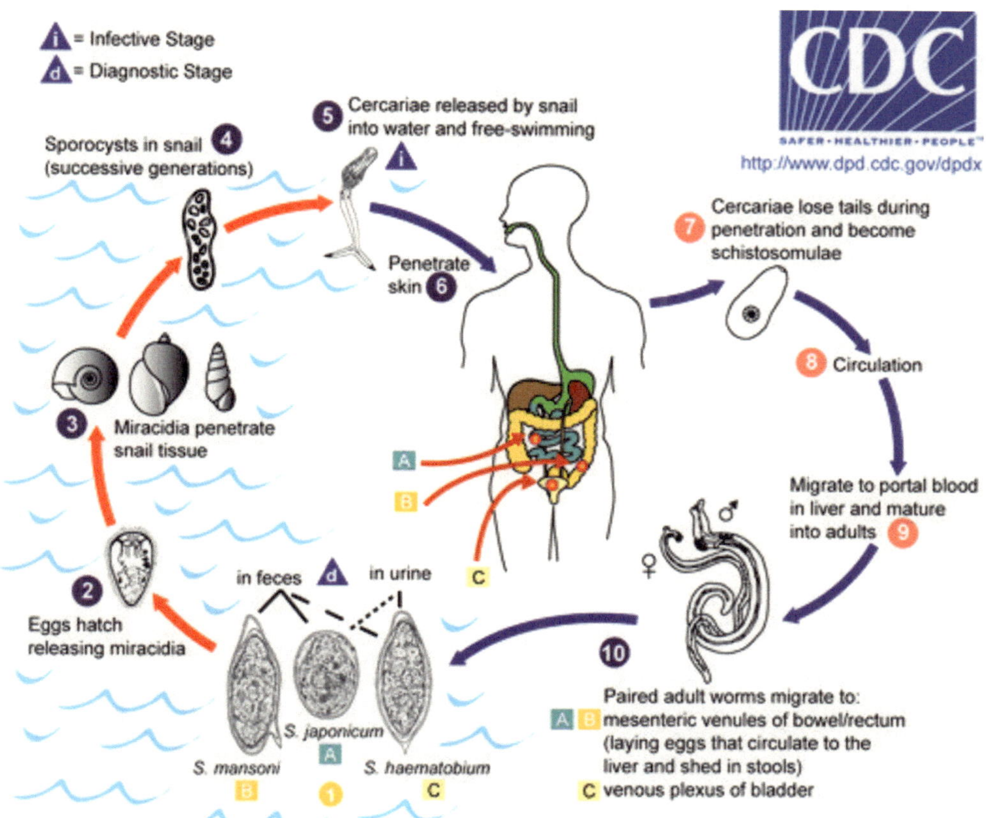

Source: Alexander J. dasilva and Melanie Moser, Public Health Image Library of the Centre for Disease Control and Prevention (CDC), USA.

Figure 1. Life cycle of schistosomes

2. Fresh water habitats harbouring snail hosts of schistosomes

Fresh water habitats can be divided into six (6) main categories having the following characteristics.

Shallow Pools: These are temporary rain filled depressions, approximately 0.5m in depth, frequently with a low electric conductivity and no aquatic vegetation. Substrate may be laterite, topsoil, sand or even granite. **Excavations**: These include borrow pits formed during road construction and deep, hand dug excavations. It is devoid of vegetation and has low conductivity. The substrates include laterite or sandy subsoil. It retains water after rains.

Small earth dam: Consist of impoundments of seasonal streams with sparse vegetation.

River and Marshes: They are characterized by having fringing hydrophytic flora and gentle flow. They are perennial, their water supply being regulated by dams.

Irrigation Channels: The substances are concrete or clay. The channels are frequently colonized by aquatic flora such as *Typhaipomoea* and *sedges.*

Reservoirs and Lakes: These are major habitats ranging in surfaces from 10 ha – 17000 ha. They undergo marked seasonal and long-term changes in water level. The aquatic vegetation is poor, the main colonizing plant being *Typha*

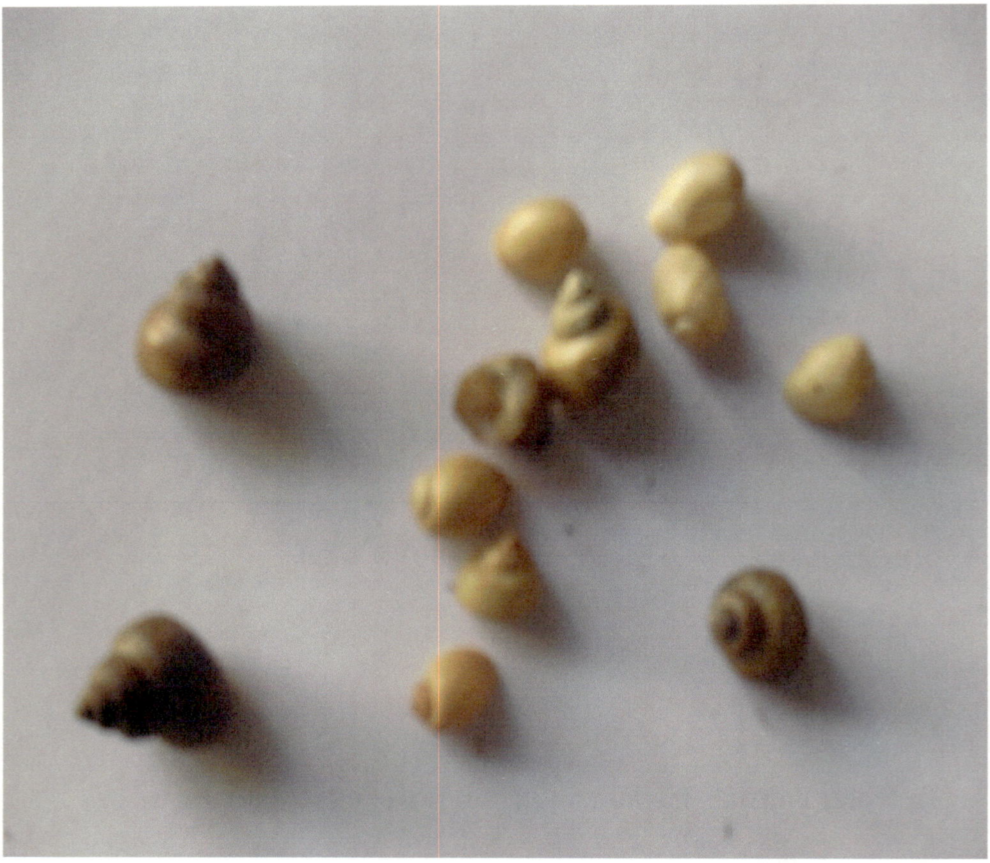

Figure 2. Shell of a host snail (*B.globosus*) ©

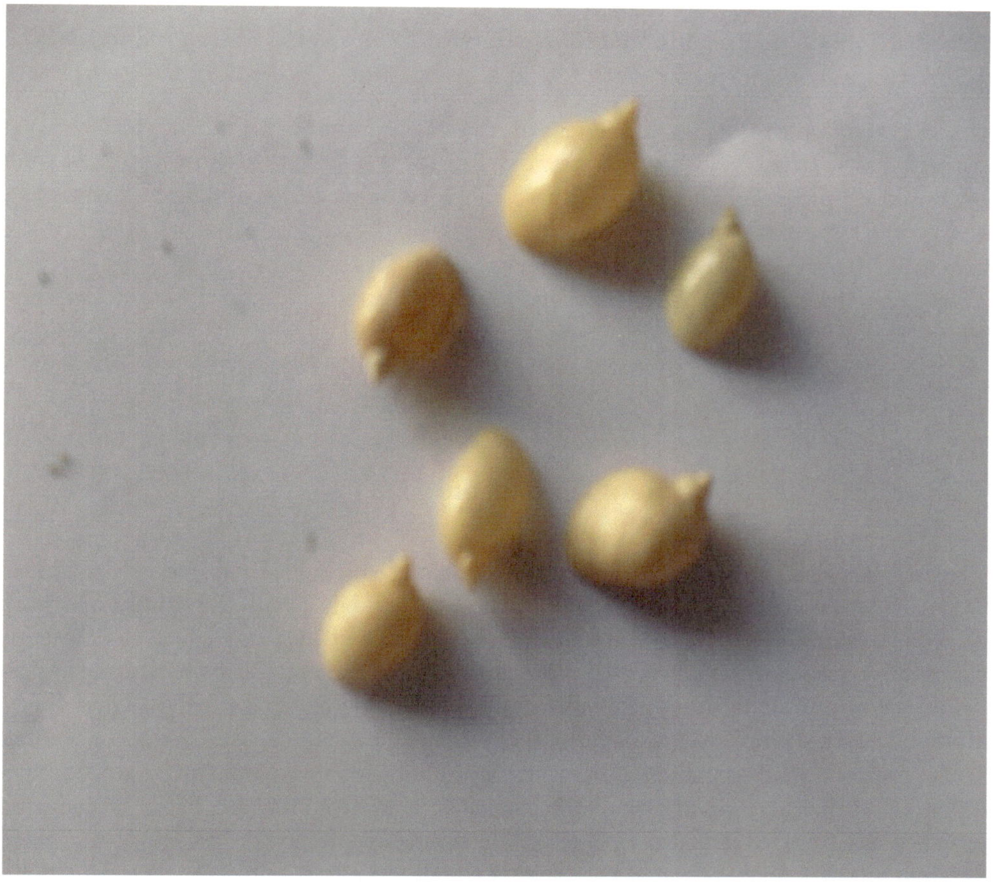

Figure 3. Shell of a host snail (*B.rohlfsi*) ©

3. Danger of schistosomiasis

Schistosomiasis cannot be eradicated worldwide at this time; neither will many of these diseases be cured by sophisticated health care services, epitomized by medical technology and large hospitals due to the insidious and complex nature of the disease. Instead the development process itself will perpetuate them [2, 3]. Irrigation projects-designed to increase the standard of living, agricultural production to improve quality of life are often planned in or near breeding ground for vectors of water-related diseases. For instance, the prevalence of schistosomiasis in many areas around the Aswan Dam in Egypt tripled after a constant bed of slow-moving water in open irrigation channels was provided for the snail – an intermediate host for the disease. However, a safe adequate water supply is generally associated with a healthier population. When Japan installed water supplies in 30 rural areas, for example, the number of cases of intestinal diseases there was reduced by 72% - (a rather substantial decrease) showing that schistosomiasis may be curtailed in endemic areas when major improvements in the standard of living have been introduced together with control of snails and reduction in both water contamination and contact.

Focus and attention on the new challenges in control programmes for schistosomiasis as well as priority research areas in the new century include: (1) status of schistosomiasis control programme; (2) progress in applied field research; (3) biology and control approaches of snail host; (4) novel approaches for schistosomiasis control; (5) pathogenesis and mobility of the disease; (6) immunology and vaccine development; (7) screening of population for chemotherapy in low transmission areas; (8) sustainable intervention methods in different endemic settings; (9) impact of animal schistosomiasis on agricultural development and importance of its control; (10) GIS/RS application and environmental changes that are very essential (3).

4. Continental distribution of schistosomiasis

Epidemiology of schistosomiasis refers to the prevalence, incidence and intensity of infection by a particular schistosome in man or animal. The prevalence rate gives the proportion of subjects who are infected at a given point in time, while intensity of infection" is a measure of vector burden of a subject or a group of subjects. On the other hand, the incidence rate indicates the proportion of initially uninfected subjects who become infected during a given period. Within an endemic area, focal transmission of schistosomiasis, whether human or animal, is the most common while prevalence and intensity of infection vary widely from one locality to another (4). Studies of the distribution of *S. haematobium* showed that it could be endemic with prevalence rate of up to 85%. Prevalence of infection is usually lower in those areas closer to the main roads than farther away, a pattern that usually coincides with urbanization including but not limited to the distribution of piped water.

A previous cross-sectional epidemiological survey on intestinal schistosomiasis due to *Schistosoma mansoni* in Wondo Genet, Southern Ethopia in 1999 was made to generate pre-intervention parasitological and malacological baseline data to be used as a reference in evaluation of community-based pilot control trial. The data obtained showed that for a total of 3000 stool specimens, collected from school children enrolled in 14 schools and microscopically examined using Kato method, the overall prevalence and intensity of *Schistosomiasis mansoni* was 34.6% and 184 eggs per grain of stool (EPG) respectively. Children excreting *Schistosoma mansoni* eggs were found in all of the 14 schools surveyed with a prevalence of infection ranging from 1.9% in one school to 80.6% in another. The overall prevalence of *S. mansoni* infection among males and females was 38.4% and 27.3%, respectively (P=0.0001. 95% C.I = 7.5% - 14.7%) whereas the intensity of infection was 186 EPG and 181 EPG, respectively (P = 0.8045, 95 and C.I = 1.17% - 1.23%). Malacological surveys of 27 water contact sites revealed the occurrence of *Biomphalaria pfeifferi* in 8 sites out of which 3 harboured infected snails shedding Schistosoma cercariae. The result shows the necessity of initiating community-based sustainable control programme. Similarly, (6) carried out a study on the feasibility and effectiveness of introducing active teaching methods into primary schools in Tanzania with a view to enhancing health education. The focus was on personal hygiene with reference to the control of schistosomiasis and helminth infections. In a randomly selected group of children compared with a comparison group, there was evidence of changes in both knowledge and health seeking behavior. In a survey of urinary schistosomiasis and trichomoniasis conducted among 830 inhabitants of Ikao village, in Owan Local Government area of Edo State, Nigeria between October 1999 and February 2000, 178 (21.4%) of subjects excreted *Schistosoma haematobium* ova in-their urine. School children were more infected than the farmers and petty traders who unlike the school children do not arbitrarily get into water contact, thus showing the importance of health education and personal hygiene. Males were noticed to be more infected than females. Most of the inhabitants had infection, while in all, urinary schistosomiasis and trichomoniasis co-infection occurred in the genito-urinary tract of 14 (6.3%) female inhabitants.

Information on the prevalence of morbidity is needed for re-calculation of the Global Burden of disease (WHO) due to *Schistosomiasis*. The data describes expression related to logistic regression including associations between prevalence of infection and prevalence of early morbidity (diarrhea, blood in stool and abdominal pain), hepatosplenic morbidity and later morbidity (haematemesis and ascitis). Diarrhoea, blood in stool due to *S. mansoni* infection mainly occurs in communities with a high prevalence of infection. The construction of George dams and reservoirs with changes in environmental conditions will influence the chances for schistosome infection to human and animals to a high level. However, the most important factor in the epidemiology of schistosomiasis is the common daily activities of villagers living in the endemic areas which constitute the risk factors for infection. Severe disease is associated with advanced infection status with signs and symptoms of portal hypertension dominating the clinical situations, and death is usually due to bleeding from ruptured esophageal varices [6, 7, 8,9]

4.1. Advancement in methodologies for schistosomiasis survey

Recent advances in schistosomiasis epidemiological surveys have resulted in the development of models such as Geographic information system (GIS) risk models for the snail-borne diseases caused by *Schistosoma* spp. and Fasciola spp. based on climate and satellite – retrieved data on temperature and vegetation coverage, making it possible to describe a relationship between vegetation index (Normalized Differences Vegetation Index (NDVI), land surface temperature (T(max) and disease prevalence, but with little reference to the distribution of the corresponding intermediate host snail, despite it is a key factor determining distribution of the disease in sub-Saharan Africa. Indeed a good snail distribution mode would probably mirror the endemic area of schistosomiasis. Snail distribution data corresponds with schistosomiasis prevalence data in relation to a forecast model based on NDVI and T (max) data derived from the Advanced Very High Resolution Radiometer (AVH RR) on board the National Oceanic and Atmospheric Administration Satellite Series. The 'best fit' model included NDVI values from 125 to 145 and a T (max) data range of 10-32 degrees C. These model included 92.3, 90.4 and 94.6% of the positive snail sample sites in GIS query overlay areas extracted from annual, dry season and wet season composite maps, respectively in Ethopia. For other sites in Africa, other NDVI and T (max) ranges may be more appropriate, depending on the species of snails present.

Similarly, In a 4 year study a geographic information system (GIS) risk model for predicting the relative risk of schistosomiasis in Kafr Elsheikh governorate, Egypt was constructed. The model, using data collected on snail population bionomics-infection rates, water quality, underground water table and cercariometry at 13 hydrologically representative sites enabling the study of role of soil type, water table and water quality at 79 of 154 rural health unit sites, validated previous models. The model permitted retrieval of relevant data by RHU 10 (rural health unit) point location. The model for the first time in Egypt supported Ministry of Health efforts to make more accurate control programme decisions based on environmental predilection sites of endemic *Schistosoma mansoni*. The possible utilization of acute phase proteins (APPs) in predicting severity of urinary schistosomiasis among infected subjects has also been canvassed.

Presently, there is a global network for the control of snail borne diseases using satellite surveillances and GIS. It came from a team residency sponsored by the Rockefeller Foundation in Bellagio, Italy, 10-14 April 2000, where an organizational plan was conceived to create a global network of collaborating health workers and earth scientists dedicated to the development of computer–based models that can be used for improved control programs for schistosomiasis and other snail-borne diseases of medical and veterinary importance. The models consist of GIS methods; global climate model data, sensor data from earth observing satellites, disease prevalence data, distribution and abundance of snail hosts, and digital maps of key environmental factors that affect development and propagation of snail-borne disease agents. The collaboration plan calls for linking a 'central resource group' at the World Health Organization, the Food and Agricultural organization, Louisiana State University and the Danish Bilharzias Laboratory with regional GIS networks to be initiated in East Africa, South Africa, West Africa, Latin America and South Asia. An Internet site, www.gnosis GIS. Org (GIS Network on Snail borne infections with special reference to schistosomiasis) has been initiated to allow interaction of team members as a "virtual research group". The sites point users to a tool box of common resources resident on computer at member organizations, provide assistance on routine use of GIS health maps in selected national disease control programme and provide a forum for development projects and climate variation and the advancement through computerized models such as Remote Sensing (RS) by earth observing satellite, a technology particularly well suited to pinpointing constraining endemic factors. Imaging techniques such as ultrasonography echo Doppler cardiography, computerized tomography (CT scan) and Magnetic Resonance Imaging (MRI) introduced a new perspective, and expanded our knowledge on morbidity [10,11, 12,13,14].

4.2. Morbidities associated with schistosomiasis

Three well-defined syndromes caused by *Schistosomiasis infections* have been revealed. The syndromes are the stage of invasion, acute schistosomiasis (katayama fever), and chronic schistosomiasis. The complications of the acute and chronic syndromes have also been reported, namely pulmonary hypertension, neuroschistosomiasis, association with salmonella, and association with staphylococci, viral hepatitis B and glomerulonephritis. In most individuals with hepatosplenic schistosomiasis the spleen is increased in size. Intestinal schistosomiasis in individuals with low worm burdens is very difficult to diagnose and therefore laborious to control. There is strong epidemiologic evidence linking *Schistosoma haematobium* infection with carcinoma of the bladder, the utility of cytological screening for urinary tract cancer has not been critically evaluated in *S. haematobium* – endemic populations. *S. haematobium* infection is regarded to be associated with increased risk for cytological abnormality such as metaplasia and hyper keratosis. Correlation exists between metaplasia and *S. haematobium* infection prevalence early in life. Morbidity results from granulomatous response to *S mansoni* eggs deposited in peripheral portal veins.

The resurgence and emergence of old and new infectious diseases in twenty first century is a major source of morbidity and mortality. Recent among these are HIV/AIDS, hanta virus pulmonary syndrome, lyme disease, haemolytic uremic syndrome, rift valley fever, dengue haemorrhagic fever, malaria, cryptosporidiosis and schistosomiasis. Related to this are the treatment modalities which include permissive use of antibiotics, the industrial use of antibiotics, demographic changes, social behavior patterns, changes in ecology, global warming and the inability to deliver minimal healthcare and the neglect of well established public health priorities that is a source of major concern globally. Since the distribution of schistosomiasis is focal, then if the resources available for control are to be used most effectively, they need to be directed towards the individuals and/or communities at highest risk of morbidity from schistosomiasis [15, 16].

5. Approaches in schistosomiasis control

The use of chemotherapy plays a leading role in the control of schistosomiasis. Snail control by the use of molluscicides is being explored in integrated control programmes. The level of effectiveness of this method however, is still subjective.It has been shown that male and female schistosomes' exhibit regional and sexual differences in susceptibility to chemotherapy that represent a form of evasive strategy of the parasite. The control of schistosomiasis therefore by molluscicides is linked to the interdependence of immunotherapy and chemotherapy. Mass chemotherapy alone in regions of high prevalence, may provide good results initially, but it might be unable to give a lasting effect due to great environmental variations., hence, the need for back up approaches such as snail control.

For snail control, molluscicides such as frescon, sodium penta chlorophenate, organotin, dinitrophenol, carbamates, niclosamide and copper sulphate are effective against aquatic and amphibious snails and their eggs.

Combining low doses of praziquantel and oxamniquine (⅓ the curative dose of praziquantel plus ⅓ the curative dose of oxamniquine) for instance can result in potentiating effect in animals receiving combination therapy. Also low concentration of aridanin (0.25 mg/ml) reduced the production of cercariae by snails already shedding cercariae. Aridanin and Aridan both produced profound reduction in the worm recovery of mice infected with pretreated cercariae of *S. mansoni* and *S. bovis*, showing its efficacy at reducing the transmission of schistosomiasis at different stages of the schistosome development.

It has been reported that snails infected with *S. mansoni* and *S. bovis* and fed with a food - praziquantel mixture - stopped shedding cercariae for several days. Histological studies showed that at the exact moment of this treatment, there was a total destruction of many nearly mature cercariae. But it has also been shown that through genetic crosses between phenotypically resistant and sensitive schistosomes' resistance to hycanthone and oxamniquine by schistosomes is a common occurrence and that it behaves like a recessive trait, thus suggesting that resistance is due to the lack of some factors. Presently, advocacy is for the appropriate application of a schistosomal vaccine, which when it becomes available will expedite the eradication of this parasite infecting greater than 200 million people and livestock [17, 18].

6. Survey, identification and distribution of species of snail hosts, in Nigeria

Certain species of African fresh water snails are exceedingly important both from a medical and veterinary viewpoint. However, there is dearth of literature through which these snails can be identified in a reliable manner according to species. This is so as more species are still being discovered. Snails' species are however identifiable using criteria spelt out in the bulletin published by WHO snail identification center, Danish Bilharziasis Laboratory. The bulletin is a field guides to African fresh water snails [19, 20]. Snails of interest could be identified by the following criteria:

Bulinus rohlfsi (Clessin):

It is usually 11 x 7.7mm when fully matured but frequently smaller. The shell is usually very light, almost white and with a low spire. The distinctly arrowhead shaped mesocone of the lateral teeth only partially separated from the endocone.

Bulinus globosus (Morelet):

It is usually in the range of 16 x 12mm and 22.5 x 14mm but sometimes larger. The distinctive character is the copulatory organ with a vergic sheath, which is not wider than preputium.

With a few exceptions all mollusks of medical or veterinary importance live in fresh water. According to their great age, several of the families have an almost worldwide distribution. Some are represented on all continents while others are missing only in South America or Australia. Others are only known from the tropics but then, as a rule, are found in the New as well as the Old World. Almost all members of one and the same family of fresh water mollusks are often to great extent alike, no matter from where in the world they descend [21,22].

The determination of species is often a very difficult problem, and without sufficient experience with regard to the family and country in question, correct identification is almost impossible except by the use of good field guide. This is due to two factors, i.e. partly the great variability found within most freshwater mollusks and partly the lack of good distinctive characters. *B. globosus* is an infrequent species in Kano State, being found in well established rain pools and restricted to the South of the 12^0 parallel. It is present in Borno State. The distribution of *B. rohlfsi* is widely reported in Kano and in Ibadan and Akure in South West, Nigeria [23, 24] and in area such as Epe in Lagos State.

In these areas, temporary water bodies (being tropical zone) are the principal foci of transmission of schistosomiasis in humans. Perennial habitats were important transmission sites that represent only a small portion of the overall problem [25].

7. Ecological factors affecting intermediate snail hosts

A combination of both abiotic and biotic factors exert their influences on the fecundity and hence population density of snails in a given habitat. The effects of the two are interrelated and are discussed in the following sections.

7.1. Fresh water malacology

With a few exceptions, all mollusks of medical or veterinary importance live in fresh water. Through familiarity with the snails and bivalves within a certain area, mere looking at the shell can help determine from which lake or river an individual snail originates. This is due to the fresh water mollusks being influenced to a high degree by the environment under which they live. Most fresh water mollusks prefer stagnant or slowly running water. On the exposed shores of big lakes and in fast-flowing rivers there are few if any pulmonates whereas prosobranchs and bivalves may be present. They are usually lacking in very acid or alkaline water, but apart from these exceptions they can be found in all types of freshwater bodies from the greatest lakes to small rainwater pools. In great lakes they are most plentiful in sheltered bays with shallow water, but sometimes they live at greater depths, down to 10 meters or more for pulmonates and 150 – 200 meters for prosobranchs and bivalves. When these snails are absent at greater depths, the reason is lack of oxygen [26,27].

According to this report, smaller lakes, ponds, and sluggish streams are the preferred habitat for most of the species. Presence of water lilies, as a rule is indicative of good conditions for snail life while Nile lettuce seems to indicate poor conditions. Papyrus swamps are also regarded as bad habitats. Certain species of freshwater pulmonates (snails) are known to live preferably or entirely in temporary pools, even in pools that hold water during only a few months of the year. It is known that many populations of fresh water pulmonates are subjected to great fluctuations, which means that species abundant at one visit might seem to be very scarce a few months later. Repeated visits are therefore advised to be sure that all species have been found, even in small ponds. It has been noted that temporary water bodies in the tropical zone are the principal foci of transmission of schistosomiasis in humans. Perennial habitats are regarded as important transmission sites that represent only a small portion of the overall problem.

8. Habitat water chemistry parameters, snail's availability and spread

Although the influence and effect of ecological physico-chemical properties of fresh water (water chemistry) on snails availability, distribution and survival is in no doubt, yet no clear picture has emerged on the overall influence they exert. Usually a very few distinct relationships exist in snail ecology and there is a general lack of precise data. It is very difficult to define and evaluate the significance of an individual environmental factor- whether physical, chemical or biological when all may be mutually affecting one another and their combined effect influencing a particular species or population. Fresh water snails are capable of adapting to wide range of environmental conditions such as water bodies with moderate organic content, little turbidity and substratum rich in organic matter and moderate light [28]. It is known that major changes in patterns of transmission (i.e. availability of infected snail hosts) occur after man-made disturbances of the ecosystem, whether by physical or chemical changes to the environment. Works on the chemistry of water in different snail habitats (29, 30, 31) in Nigeria and other countries indicate that most snails are tolerant of water differing greatly in chemical content.

An outbreak of intestinal schistosomiasis reported at Richard – Toll, 130km from the dam of Diama, Senegal, was the first sign that the ecological changes caused by the dam had an impact on the prevalence of schistosomiasis. Since the main functions of the Diama dam were prevention of seawater intrusion, provision of a reservoir of fresh water for irrigation and domestic supply of water for municipal use in Dakar, it was suspected that it was likely that the dam induced both physical and chemical environmental changes. In addition to increasing the number of water bodies around the area, the Diama dam prevented salt-water intrusion into the river and the marigots of the Delta, thereby creating new habitats in areas previously unsuitable for fresh water snails [31].

In July 1983, salinities as high as 19.9% were recorded in the Senegal River at Richard – Toll [32,33] showed that the dam caused a gradual softening of the Lac de Guiers water: water mineralization has decreased 20% in the Northern part and nearly 50% in the Southern region. At the same time the formerly important yearly variations in salinity have distinctly diminished. However, because of the dearth or non availability of physical or chemical data from selected transmission sites at that time, it was concluded that it will be difficult predicting how the expected ecological changes influence snail habitats, especially since it is usually not possible to predict colonization of a particular habitat through chemical analysis of its water content. Interesting results have been obtained showing that the hatchability of eggs, the fecundity and survival of adult *B. africanus* had been adversely affected by salinities as low as 1.0%, with the most significant reductions occurring between 3.5% and 4.5% [34]. From other recent studies it also appeared that trematode parasitism reduces the salt tolerance of the snail intermediate hosts. A decrease in hatching of schistosome ova with increasing salinity has also been observed. Poor survival of *B globosus* hatchings in water with a conductivity of 125μs is known. *B. truncatus* is adapted to hard water, in contrast to *Biomphalaria* sp. Another indication that salinity may have been one of the major reasons for the low prevalence of schistosomiasis in the Senegal River Basin Delta (SRB) was the existence of an endemic focus for *S. haematobi-*

um infections in a village of Lampsar, 20km from the Atlantic Ocean. There *B. Senegalensis* and *B. globosus* were the likely intermediate hosts for *S. haematobium*. The probable reason for the presence of these bulinid species was the existence for a long time (more than 50 years) of several barrages on the Lampsar River that prevented salt intrusion from the Senegal River. There is, however, conflicting evidence on the role of salinity. The spreading of *B globosus* in the Lampsar River is said to be linked to more stable levels of water bodies and increased irrigation channels rather than reduced levels of salinity. In contrast, in the transmission sites directly associated with water bodies in the Delta, reduction in salinity may play a role in further spread of schistosomiasis. Thus, due to all these ecological changes, areas previously unsuitable for fresh water snails are now providing ideal habitats. The results of these changes are not only increases in the size of existing snail populations, but also spread and colonization of these new habitats by other bulinid species. Influences from the parameters from various types of snail habitats in SRB (Senegal River Basin) showed no significant variations in values between the dry and rainy season except that temperatures were higher in the month of October; but pH and conductivity remained within the levels of tolerance for bulinids. Although the focal distribution of schistosomiasis is linked to water resources development, the factors contributing to local variations in prevalence and intensities of infection are not yet understood. No evidence in the Transvaal supported claiming that the chemical composition of natural unpolluted water plays any part in determining vector snail habitats but that pollutions (such as the presence of sewage or industrial wastes) and turbidity appear to have adverse effects on bilharziasis vectors. Long term population fluctuations are greatly affected by spates (flooding) associated with heavy rainfall, which of course will increase the turbidity of the water bodies so affected. In the model developed, they observed the population dynamics of the fresh water snail *B globosus* such as abundance changes, recruitment rates, and mortality rates for adult snails in river habitats in Zimbabwe was such that the rate of recruitment into the adult population is dependent on temperature, incorporating a time lag to allow for growth to adult size using the mathematical model. It has been observed that the flood that was likely to occur as a result of constructions of three (3) George Reservoirs in Yangtze, China which could interfere with the development of snails, with the flushed beaches and migratory settlements at certain attitude becoming snail habitats, making the reservoir area, a potential transmission area of schistosomiasis due to dispersal of infectious resources. Also in a UNDP/ WORLD BANK/WHO special programme for Research and training in Tropical Diseases results showed that climates and topography effectively restrict vector –borne infections to certain geographical areas, a clear illustration of how strongly the spatial distributions of these diseases rely on environmental factors. This then call for detailed study and analysis of various physico-chemical parameters in snail ecological habitats, for the purpose of better understanding of how the diseases they transmit could be checked effectively.

8.1. pH of water bodies

Low pH could be harmful to snails. This is due to the possibility of denaturation of the mucus on the exposed skin surface; extremes of pH i.e. low as well very high pH will be harmful to these snails as both could denature the glyco proteins (mucus) on their exposed skin surface.

8.2. Alkalinity

This refers to the (carbonate) CO_3^{2-} and (bicarbonate) HCO_3^- content in the water bodies. Concentration of 50mg/L is regarded as weak, 100 mg/L as medium while 200mg/L is regarded as strong (34,35).

8.3. Total Dissolved Solids (TDS)

The presence of sewage or industrial wastes in waters bodies is regarded as an important factor in determining vector snail habitats, as they constitute pollutions and snails could only adapt to water bodies with moderate organic content. Water bodies may contain suspended solids, inorganic, organic chemicals, biodegradable organic matter, pathogenic microorganisms, and metals. Pathogenic microorganisms and indicator pathogens are found in high concentrations per gram of raw sewage, and if allowed to accumulate and sit, untreated water produces malodorous emissions as a result of decomposition of organic material.

Solids in water bodies are usually measured as solid, total and dissolved total solids. A typical water body contains solids, total as 350mg/L (Weak), 720 mg/L (Medium) and 1,200mg/L (Strong) while TDS in the range of 250mg/L (Weak); 500mg/L (Medium) and 850 mg/L (Strong) [35,36].

8.4. Color

Pure water is colorless but the presence of pollutions in water bodies give rise to varied colors. It has been observed that vector snails appeared to prefer clean, clear water bodies to colored water [24].

8.5. Turbidity

Snail vectors are generally intolerant of high turbidities. Intermediate host snails found in most cases in naturally turbid water tend to decrease as the turbidity of the habitat pool increase. It has also been shown that while a turbidity of 360mg/L (due to suspended mineral from granite erosion) did not affect snails themselves, it prevented development and hatching of *B. pfeifferi* eggs [37]. It was noted that both *B. globosus* and *Lymndea natalensis* are tolerant to this concentration of suspended particles as their eggs hatch normally at a level of 190mg/L. The water composition of most snail habitats is usually eutropic, having some dissolved organic materials showing that snails are negatively affected by turbid water.

8.6. Total hardness

This is indicated by the total concentration of Ca^{2+} and Mg^{2+} ions present in water bodies, different concentrations of calcium and magnesium ions affect the mortality rates of snails while egg production by *B. pfeifferi* kept in both natural streams and artificial culture medium with high magnesium (Mg^{2+}) and Ca^{2+}) ratios (12:4 and 19:7 respectively) is usually reduced. *B. truncatus* is adapted to hard water, in contrast to *B. pfeifferi*. This fact may help to explain the reason why *B. truncatus* was fairly widespread in the Delta (Senegal River Basin) prior to the building of the Diama dam. The existence of a relationship between the occurrence of *B. pfeifferi* and *B. globosus* and low stretches of watercourses over rocks with hardness of 5 or more in Mohs' scale of hardness in the South –eastern Transvaal, suggesting adverse effects of hard water on the thriving of snail hosts.

8.7. Chloride ion (Cl^-)

The concentration of this ion is a measure of salinity of a particular water body. Salinity has been reported to exert great influence on the availability of vector snails in a given habitat. The hatchability of eggs and the fecundity and survival of adult *B. Africanus* had been adversely affected by salinities as low as 1.0% with the most significant reductions occurring between 3.5% and 4.5%, salinity even in low value plays a major role in the low prevalence of schistosomiasis in Senegal River Basin Delta, where the construction work brought about reduction in salinity resulting in new outbreaks of both intestinal and urinary schistosomiasis in the area. A decrease in hatching of schistosome eggs with increasing salinity has also been observed. Concentration of 30mg/L is regarded as weak, 50mg/L as medium and 100 mg/L as strong [34,35].

9. Study sites

Fresh water bodies namely: Kanye and Rimin Gado dams (Kano), Lagoon front (Unilag, Akoka, Lagos) and Oyan dam (Ogun-Osun river basin, Abeokuta) were surveyed for 3 years.

Two snail species (*Bulinus globosus and Bulinus rohlfsi*) were searched for and collected quarterly (May – August and November –February) in these sites because they are established sites for these snails. However, this is the first time the presence of these snails will be reported at the Lagoon front, University of Lagos.

9.1. Kanye and Rimin Gado

Kanye is a small village, located about 45km west of Kano city. The Kanye dam is about 600 x 800 m in size, with a shallow flat and steep margin and 100% exposure to sunlight. The vegetation consists of the aquatic plant *Chara sp*, which grows luxuriously during the dry season. Also present, is the aquatic flora, *sedges* and waterweeds, dense *Najas sp*. and moderate *Typha sp*. The snail species such as *B. rohlfsi*, *B. globosus* and *Biomphalaria pfeifferi* are abundant in Kanye and Rimin Gado dams, which serve as a major domestic source of water supply to the inhabitants, as only few public taps, which do not run regularly, are available. Laundry, bathing and cattle grazing are pronounced around the dam. The second dam, located at Rimin Gado and designated as Kanye II is located some 20km West of Kano city. The dam is a reservoir of a shallow impoundment of a small seasonal river. It is about 500m x 800m in size. The exposure of the surface to sunlight is 100%. The substrate is a fine sandy soil, topped by a thin layer of clay and humus. It has the same vegetational features as Kanye (I) and contains same snail species. Human interference through laundry, bathing, farming and animal grazing is very prominent.Species of *B. globosus and B. rohlfsi* were collected there and water samples were taken.

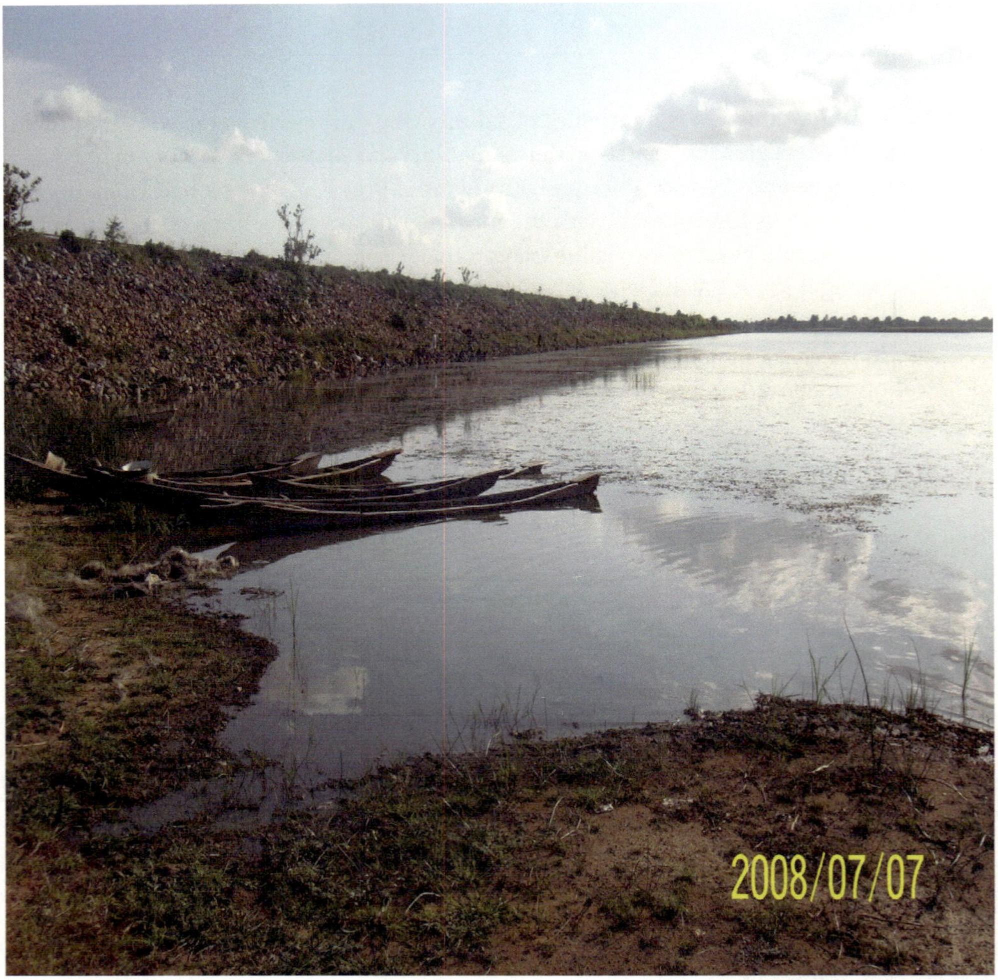

Figure 4. Rimin Gado dam, Rimin Gado area, Kano, Kano state, Nigeria.

9.2. Lagoon front, University of Lagos

The Akoka Campus of the University of Lagos, an area of about 320 hectares located in the North East of Yaba Lagos, was a part of study area. Acquired in 1962, the acquisition notice gave the extent as 807 acres. The 320 hectares of the University of Lagos Land comprises of 174 hectares of good building ground and 146 hectares of swamp or swampy area. The swamps are divided into the northern swamp which covers an area of 61 hectares, eastern swamp 24 hectares, southern swamp 40 hectares and the center – finger swamps 16.5 hectares.

The Akoka Campus of the University of Lagos is located on latitude of 6°22′N – 6° 44′N and longitude of 3° 29′E. It is bounded in the west by the Ogbe River (traversed by a bridge between Abule Oja and the main gate of the University), in the North by Akoka Ilaje, in the South by Iwaya and East by the Lagos Lagoon.

The campus being located in the center of Lagos has the same climate as Lagos. The climate of Lagos is of the equatorial type. All the year round, temperature is usually above 65°F and average 85°F. There is minimal seasonal variation of about 10°F between the hottest month (March) and the coolest month (August). Relative humidity is usually between 80% and 100% dropping to about 70% in the afternoon during the dry season. April to October marks the extent of the rainy season with an average annual rainfall of 1830mm. Despite the relative flatness of the area, spatial variation is great.

9.3. Oyan Dam (Ogun-Osun river basin authority, Abeokuta)

The Oyan Reservoir is located on Latitude 7° 14″ N and Longtitude 3° 13″ E, at an elevation of 43.3 m above sea level. It has a catchment area of approximately 9000km^2 within the southern climatic belt of Nigeria. The belt is characterized by a rainy season of about eight months (March – October) and a dry season of about four months (November – February); a mean annual precipitation of 1000 – 1250 mm a mean relative humidity of 75% - 100% and a mean annual temperature of about 30°C.

The soil is generally composed of crystalline acid rocks of the ferruginous tropical type that have been moderately to strongly leached with low humus content. It is characterized by weak acidic to neutral surface layers and moderately to strongly acid sub-layers. The area falls within the 'Ibadan Group' which overlies the metamorphic rocks of the basement complex [38].

The vegetation is mainly savanna of the low forest type. This is characterized by sparsely distributed short trees in a predominantly grass land, as a result of timber lumbering, bush burning and cultivation of an original rain forest.

10. Methods

10.1. Collection and selection of experimental snail samples

10.1.1. Procedures

Snail sampling for species of *Bulinus globosus* and *Bulinus rohlfsi* was carried out quarterly (May – August and November - February) during dry and rainy seasons using standard technique involving drag scoop supplemented by manual search. The contents of the scoop were searched by visual inspection and by inspection of the underside of boats, bamboo rafts, floating and submerged sticks and vegetation. All snails collected from each station (i.e. scoop and manual searches) were pooled and recorded as number of snails per site per quarter. All snails were identified (Tables 1 and 2).

Dam	*B. globosus*	*B. rohlfsi*
Rimin Gado & Kanye	293	450
Oyan	259	83
Lagoon front	158	0
TOTAL	710	533

Table 1. Total Snail catch from the study sites surveyed.

Parameter	Kanye Dam		Rimin Gado Lake		Lagoon Front		Oyan Dam	
Snail species	*Glob*	*Rohl*	*Glob*	*rohl*	*Glob*	*rohl*	*Glob*	*rohl*
Snail catch	188.0	340.0	105.0	110.0	158.0	0.0	259.0	83.0
PH at 25ºC	7.2	7.3	7.2	5.6	5.9	6.9	5.6	7.5
Total alkalinity (CaCO3) (mg /L)	120.0	120.0	218.0	209.6	108.	180.0	47.0	49.0
Total dissolved solids (TDS) (mg/L)	158.4	160.2	596.6	618.8	296.4	301.2	205.8	208.2
Total Hardness (mg/L)	47.0	49.2	66.8	96.9	96.0	87.4	13.3	13.5
Calcium (mg/L)	40.0	42.0	29.3	30.2	32.4	28.9	7.6	7.5
Magnesium (mg/L)	7.0	7.2	37.5	66.7	63.6	58.5	5.7	6.0
Salinity (%)	14.3	13.9	14.7	14.1	27.8	28.1	2.8	2.6
Turbidity (m)	5.2	5.0	4.2	6.8	3.6	3.7	1.0	0.9
Colour (NTU)	10	10	15.0	25.0	10.0	15.0	10.0	10.0
Biochemical Oxygen demand (BOD) (mg/L)	5.0	5.8	19.5	20.2	14.2	14.8	5.0	4.8
Dissolved Oxygen (mg/L)	4.5	4.7	6.2	5.3	2.5	2.7	5.3	5.6

Glob: B. globosus snail caught in the surveyed water bodies

Rohl: B. rohlfsi snail caught in the survey water bodies

Table 2. The median values of some physico-chemical properties of surveyed water bodies.

11. Result

Survival of snails collected during the dry season subjected to aestivation for 30 days at 25ºC was 20 *B. globosus* out of the 30 used representing 67.0% survival and 10 dead representing 33.0%.Similarly, 16 *B. rohlfsi* representing 88% survival while 2 or 12.0% died.

26 *B. globosus* or 87% survived while 4 or 13.0% died during starvation for 30 days, while 18 or 78.3% of the 23 *B. rohlfsi* survived while 5 or 28.0% died. No mortality was recorded in the control (fed) group.

During rainy season however, 16 *B. globosus* or 94.0% survived aestivation while 14 *B. rohlfsi* or 82.0% survived 27 *B. globosus* representing 90.0% survived starvation while 23 *B. rohlfsi* representing 76.0% survived starvation respectively.

Four *B. globosus* or 4.0% that were dead in the control group while 9 *B. rohlfsi* or 10.0% were recorded dead in the control group.

B. globosus in the control group survived best followed by *B. rohlfsi* in the same group. Aestivating *B. rohlfsi* survived the least.

Surviving snails were found buried at different depths (0.2-12.0mm) in the soil mixture while their aperture were filled with mud and were deeply retracted into the shell).

Survival was better during rainy season. The ecological conditions could be more suitable during this period survival for *B.globosus* under starvation was poor during dry season compared to rainy season while both species under feeding survived best during dry season.

There was no definite pattern in the survival but it appears that survival may be indirectly related to the infection of these snails with schistosomes.

Author details

I.S. Akande[1*] and A.A. Odetola[2]

*Address all correspondence to: iakande@unilag.edu.ng or akande_idowu@yahoo.com

1 Department of Biochemistry, College of Medicine, University of Lagos, Idi-Araba, Lagos

2 Department of Biochemistry University of Ibadan, Oyo State, Nigeria

References

[1] Oyeyi, T. I, & Ndifon, G. T. (1990). A note on the post aestivation biology of *Bulinus rohlfsi* (clessin), an intermediate host of *Schistosoma haematobium* (Bilharz) in Northern Nigeria. *Trop. Med. Parasit* , 84

[2] Strickland, G. T. (1982). Schistosomiasis- A neglected Tropical Disease' (NTDs). Rev. Infect Dis. 4 (5):

[3] Martin, G. O. (2003). Ways of thinking about Water and Disease. Lead paper delivered at the annual society conference, Nigeria Society for Parasitology, NIMR, Lagos, Nigeria: , 1-11.

[4] Xiaonong, Z, Minggand, C, Mcmanus, D, & Bergquist, R. (2002). Schistosomiasis control in the 21st century. Proceedings of the International Symposium on Schistosomiasis, Shangai, July Acta Trop. (82 92): 95- 114., 4-6.

[5] Sleigh, A. C, & Mott, K. E. (1986). Schistosomiasis. In "Clinics in Tropical Medicine and communicable Diseases". Vol. I. Chp. 8.

[6] Erko, B, Medhin, G, Berhe, N, Abebe, F, Gebre-michael, T, & Gundersen, S. G. (2002). Epidemiological studies intestinal schistosomiasis in Wondo Genet, Southern Ethopia. Ethiop. Med J. , 40(1), 29-39.

[7] Lansdown, R, Ledward, A, Hall, A, Issae, W, Yona, E, Matulu, J, Miveta, M, & Kihamia, C. (2002). *Scistosomiasis helminths* infection and health education in Tanzania achieving behaviour change in primary schools. *Health Education C. Res.* , 17(4), 425-33.

[8] Nimorsi, O. P, Egwunyenga, A. O, & Bajomo, D. O. (2001). Survey of Urinary schistosomiasis and trichomoniasis in a rural community in Edo State, Nigeria. J. commun Dis. , 33(2), 96-101.

[9] Vander-werf, M. J, De Vias, S. J, Looman, C. W, Nage-ikerke, N. J, Habbema, J. D, & Engels, D. (2002). Associating Community Prevalence of *Schistosoma mansoni* infection with prevalence of signs and symptoms. *Acta Trop.* , 82(2), 127-37.

[10] Kristensen, T. K, Malone, J. B, & Carroll, J. C. (2001). Use of Satellite remote sensing and geographic information systems to model the distribution and abundance of snail intermediate hosts in Africa: a preliminary model for *Biomphalaria Pfeifferi* in Ethopia. *Acta Trop.* , 79(1), 73-78.

[11] Urbani, C, Sinoun, M, Socheat, D, Pholsena, K, Strandgard, H, Odermatt, P, & Hatz, C. (2002). Epidemiology and control of *mekongi schistosomiasis. Acta Trop.* , 82(2), 157-68.

[12] Malone, J. B, Bergquist, N, Hun, R, Bavia, O, K, & Bernardi, M, E. M. ((2001). A global network for the control of snail- borne disease using Satellite surveill.ance and geographic information systems. Acta Trop. , 79(1), 7-12.

[13] Bergquist, N. R. (2001). Vector borne parasitic diseases: new trends in data collection and risk assessment. Acta Trop. , 79(1), 13-20.

[14] Lambertucci, J, Serufo, R, Gerspacher-lara, J, C, Rayes, R, Teixeira, A, A, Nobre, R, & Antune, V. S C. M. ((2000). *Schistosoma mansoni*: assessment of morbidity before and after control. *Acta Trop.* , 77(1), 101-109.

[15] Berns, D. S, & Ragers, B. (2000). Emerging infections diseases; a cause for concern. Isr. Med. Assoc. J. , 2(12), 919-23.

[16] Utzinger, J, Goran, N, Ossey, E. K, Booth, Y. A, Traore, M, Lohourignon, M, et al. (2000). Rapid screening for *schistosoma mansoni* in Western Cote d' Ivoire using a simple school questionnaire. *Bull. World health Organ.* , 78(3), 389-98.

[17] BotrosS; Soliman, A; el- Grawhary, N et al. ((1989). Effect of combined low dose Praziquanted and Oxamniquine on different stages of schistosome maturity. Trans R. Soc Trop med. Hyg. , 83(1), 86-9.

[18] Adewumi, C. O, & Furu, P. (1989). Evaluation of aridanin, a glycoside, and Aridan, an aqueous extract of Tetrapleura fruit on *Schistosoma manosni* and *Schistosoma bovis*. J. *Ethnopharmacol.* , 27(3), 277-83.

[19] (WHO (1978 and 1979). A Field Guide to African Fresh Water Snails. WHO snail identification center Denmark: 1- 28). 1-28.

[20] WHO ((1995). Twelve programme report of the UNDP/World Bank/WHO special programme for research and training on tropical disease research(TDR) progress,, 1975-1994.

[21] Betterton, C, & Ndifon, G. T. Bassey, S. E; Tan, R, M. and Oyeyi, T. ((1988). Schistosomiasis in kano State, Nigeria. I Human infections near dam sites and the distribution and habitat preferences of potential snail intermediate hosts. Ann. Trop. Med. Parasitol, , 82(6), 561-570.

[22] Cowper, S, & Bilharziasis, G. Schistosomiasis) in Nigeria. Tropical and Geographical medicine, , 25, 105-118.

[23] Greer, G, Mimpfound, J, & Malek, l, R. E. A. ((1990). Human Schistosomiasis in Cameroon. II. Distribution of the snail hosts. Am. J. Trop. Med. Hyg. , 42(6), 573-80.

[24] WHO ((1965). Snail control in the prevalence of bilharziasis. Geneva: 225 pp WHO (1976). Surveillance of Drinking Water Quality. WHO Geneva.

[25] WHO(1981). Bull of the World Health Organization , 59(1), 115-127.

[26] Hunter, J, Rey, M, & Chu, L. K. Y.. ((1993). Parasite diseases in water resources development: the need for intersectional negotiation. Geneva: World Health Organization. , 1-152.

[27] Webbe, G. (1982). The Parasite In: Schistosomiasis Epidemiology treatment and control.P Jordan and G. Webbe (eds) Medical Books Ltd. London , 5-6.

[28] Shutte, C. H. J, & Frank, G. H. (1964). Observations on the distribution of fresh water mollusca and chemistry of the natural water in the South Eastern Transvaal and adjacent Northern Swaziland. Bull. World Health Organizations. , 30, 387-400.

[29] Goher, H. A, & Gindy, H. I. (1960 a). b). The ecology of Egyptians snail vectors of Bilharziasis and fascioliasis I : Physical factors Proc. Egypt Acad Sci., , 15, 70-86.

[30] Ndifon, G. T. (1979). Studies on the feeding biology, anatomical variation and ecology of vectors of schistosomiasis and other fresh water snails in South Western Nigeria. Ph.D thesis, University of Ibadan, Nigeria.

[31] Vercruysse, J, Southgate, V, & Rollinson, R. D. ((1994). Studies on transmission and schistosome interaction in Senegal, Mali and Zambia. Tropical and Geographical Medicine, , 46(40), 220-226.

[32] Cogels, F. X, Thiam, A, & Gac, J. Y. (1993). Premiers effect des barrages du

[33] Philippe, C. (1993). Amenagements hydro-agricoles et evolution de environment dans Lake Gorom-lampser (delta du fleuve Senegal. *ORSTOM.*

[34] Donelly, F. A, Appleton, C. C, & Schutte, C. H. (1983). The influence of salinity on the ova and miracidia of three species of schistosoma. Int. J. parasitol. , 14, 113-120.

[35] Tchobanoglous, G, & Burton, F. (1991). Waste engineering: treatment, disposal, and reuse, 3rd edition New York: Mc Graw Hill., 584-636.

[36] De-MeillonB; De-Frank, G, H and Allanson, B, R. ((1958). Some aspects of snail ecology in South Africa, WHO technical report series. Bull World health organization; , 18, 771-783.

[37] Smyth, A. J, & Montgomery, R. F. (1962). Soils and land use in central western Nigeria. 320pp. Government Printer. Ibadan

[38] Ayoade, J. O. (1982). climate. In barbour K.M.J.S. Oguntoyinbo, J.O.C. Onyemelukwe & J.C. Nwafor (eds) Nigeria in maps. Hodder & Stoughton. London , 24-25.

Chapter 3

Community-Based Control of Schistosomiasis and Soil-Transmitted Helminthiasis in the Epidemiological Context of a Large Dam in Cote D'ivoire

Nicaise Aya N'Guessan , Orsot Niangoran Mathieu,
Abé N'Doumi Noël and N'Goran Kouakou Eliézer

Additional information is available at the end of the chapter

http://dx.doi.org/10.5772/53494

1. Introduction

Parasitic diseases, among which schistosomiasis and soil-transmitted helminthiasis (ankylostosomiasis, ascariasis and trichuriasis), affect more than two billion people through the world (WHO, 2012). These diseases occur mainly in tropical regions, are real public health problems, and have a negative impact on socioeconomic development (WHO, 2008).

Côte d'Ivoire, located in West Africa, is not spared. Many parasitic diseases exist in this country. Schistosomiasis is widespread (Doumenge et al., 1987; N'Goran et al., 1997; N'Guessan et al., 2007; Raso et al., 2005; Utzinger et al., 2000; WHO, 2011) with prevalence generally higher in communities around the water projects built to solve the problems of electrical safety and / or food (Steinmann, 2006). As for soil-transmitted helminthiasis, there is very little data on the prevalence and intensity in Côte d'Ivoire. But according to the WHO, they are common throughout the territory [WHO, 2010.3]. The available data show that the prevalence of hookworm infection may reach 100% in endemic communities in Côte d'Ivoire, 71.6% of ascariasis and trichuriasis 24%. Concerning soil-transmitted helminth infections, hookworm is the main parasite of our study area with 50% prevalence and less than 10% for other affections (N'Guessan, 2003).

In this study, we seek lasting solutions to fight against schistosomiasis and soil-transmitted helminthiasis in the ecoepidemiological context of a large dam. Our results can be extrapolated in similar epidemiological settings elsewhere in Côte d'Ivoire, and other African countries. To this end, our investigations were conducted in the locality of Taabo-village straddling the area of forest and savannah woodland. The set of two areas represents 2/3 of the different vegetation types encountered in this country. Parasitological monitoring conducted, in such eco-epidemiological context, for two consecutive years of annual mass treatment revealed a high prevalence of urinary schistosomiasis among school children. Prevalence ranged from 94% to 74% at the beginning to the end (N'Goran et al., 2001). Moreover, the evaluation of reinfection of *Schistosoma haematobium* in various eco-epidemiological systems has shown that it is faster in the context of large dams. The high prevalence and limited reductions after mass treatments could be explained by the almost continuous transmission of this parasite (N'Goran et al., 2001; N'Guessan et al., 2007).

The example of Taabo-village located near the large dam Taabo where urinary schistosomiasis is a real public health problem is remarkable (N'Goran et al., 1997 and 2001). Given the importance of this disease at Taabo-village, which approach control could put important pressure on large and sustained transmission of *S. haematobium* and hope to significantly reduce the morbidity due to urinary schistosomiasis?

In this perspective, a preventive approach and the fight against disease caused by schistosomiasis and soil-transmitted helminthiasis as recommended by the World Health Organization (WHO, 2003, 2004 a and 2004b) were implemented. We believe that the communication for behavior change associated with the ongoing management could allow a significant decrease in the prevalence and morbidity of these diseases. To do so, parasitological surveys were conducted in schools before and after a control action to assess the epidemiological situation. Then, teachers and Community Health Workers (AUC) were trained to educate and support consistently the population. Finally, sociological surveys were conducted to determine the perceptions and human factors in risk associated with the endemicity of these diseases.

2. Methods

2.1. Study area

The Taabo dam is located in south-center of Côte d'Ivoire, on the river Bandama in degraded forest area. Its construction was completed in 1979 (Sellin B. and Simonkovich, 1982). It has a maximum depth of 34 m and a dam of 7.5 km long. The water reservoir is 630 million m^3 and an area of 69 km^2. It is used to generate electricity. Taabo- village is 0.5

km far from the lake (Figure 1). This study area includes 3 929 inhabitants from the database collected in 2009 by the Demographic Surveillance System of Taabo (SSD).

2.2. Parasitological surveys

From the list of the two primary schools of the study site, a school was chosen according to the largest number of students. In the selected school, about 60 students at the rate of 10 per classroom from the first year of the primary (CP1) to the last year (CM2) were selected by lottery for the baseline survey and the second survey. Participation in the study was voluntary. Parents or guardians of selected children were invited to sign a written informed consent after explanation of the objective of the study and procedures by investigators.

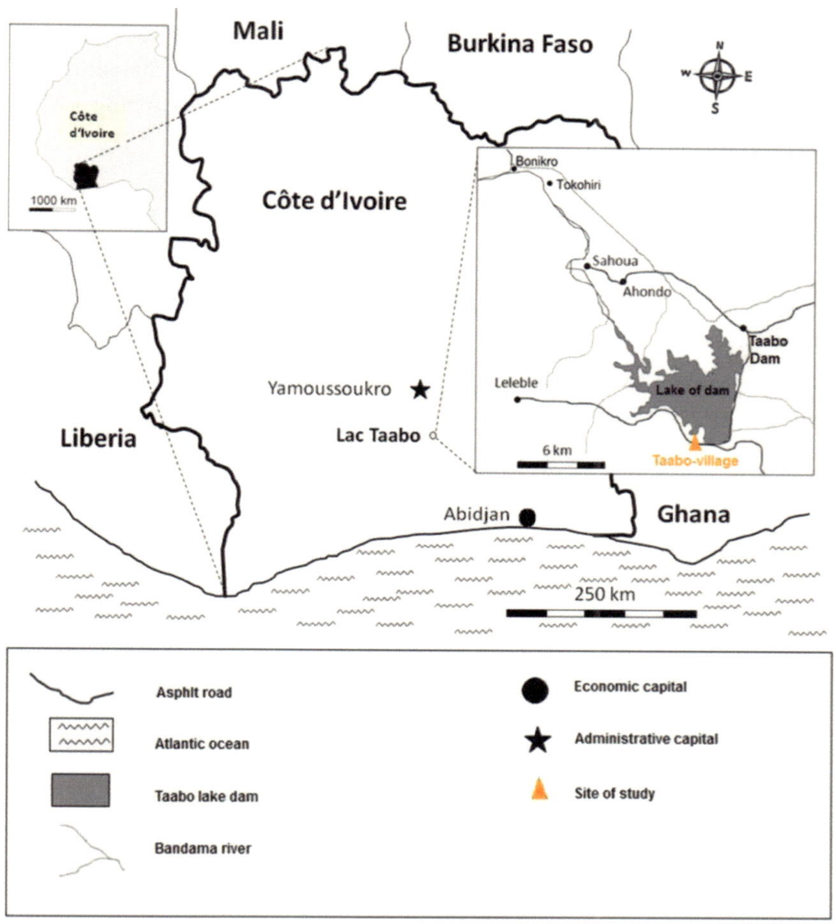

Figure 1. Overview of the study area

The selected school children participated in parasitological surveys conducted in April 2008 before treatment and on May 2009 after one year. In 2008 as in 2009, each student gave a urine sample and a stool sample. These samples were taken between 10 a.m and 2 p.m.

The search for eggs of *Schistosoma haematobium* in each urine sample was performed by the standard filtration of 10 ml of urine on a filter Nytrel ®, then the analysis of the filter under a microscope after coloration with lugol (Plouvier et al., 1975). The eggs of *Schistosoma haematobium* were identified and counted.

The stools were examined by the Kato-Katz technique, which involved analysis of 41.7 mg of stool under a microscope after plating and clarification by malachite green (Katz et al., 1972). The readings of the slides were made after 30 to 60 min for clarification in order to observe hookworms in addition to other helminths. The eggs of *Schistosoma mansoni* and soil-transmitted helminths (*Ancylostoma spp, Ascaris lumbricoides* and *Trichuris trichiura*) were detected and counted by species. The intensity of infection was expressed as number of eggs per gram of stool. After microscopic examination, a quality control was used to check the consistency of results. Prevalences and intensities of parasites were classified into three categories: mild, moderate and heavy according to WHO classification (WHO, 2004 and 2004a).

2.3. Training of teachers and community health workers (CHW) for awareness and treatment

During a workshop held in 2008 at Taabo city, two teachers and one community health worker (CHW), selected per locality and by their authorities, attended a course of half a day. They were trained to use the awareness tools and prevention on the one hand and on the other hand administration of praziquantel against schistosomiasis and mebendazole against soil-transmitted helminthiasis. Then they received the tablets, treatment forms and media for awareness and health education.

2.4. Awareness and treatment

The awareness, prevention and control studies were conducted in the two primary schools by two teachers among the school-age populations and by a CHW among the other community members. Everyone was aware of the opportunity to treat himself according to his convenience because drugs were available to them from teachers and CHW. Treatment (praziquantel and mebendazole) cost per student was 100 CFA francs in schools and 150 CFA in community during the first year. At the end of the study, all parasitized individuals were treated with praziquantel and/or mebendazole for free for ethical reasons.

2.5. Sociological survey

The sociological survey concerned on the one hand the school-age children (children attending school or not) and on the other hand the general population, particularly the heads of households. The selection of children attending school was done by a reasoned choice of 12 students per class from the first year elementary classes (CE1) to the last year of primary school (CM2). As for children who do not attend school, they have been chosen unintentionally on the ground during the investigation. Based on the estimated number of households, the quota of households to be interviewed has been determined. This survey was made after the awareness and treatment. The majority of respondents are farmers and students, the survey took place when they were free i.e in the morning (from 6:00 to 10:00) and in the evening (from 16:00 to 20:00). We collected qualitative information from focus group and quantitative information by questionnaire.

http://dx.doi.org/10.5772/53494

2.6. Data analysis

The data were analyzed using STATA software, version 9 (Stata Cooperation, College Station, Tx, USA). The various parasites were collected in two groups of diseases: schistosomiasis and soil-transmitted helminthiasis. For each condition, the prevalences and intensities of infection were calculated for each survey. the 2008 data were compared with those of 2009 by comparison test of two proportions unrelated. The treatement results of the sociological survey have been analised by the same test.

3. Results

Both parasitological surveys were conducted in Taabo-village 1 primary school, successively in 2008 and 2009. The age group of school children who participated in the survey is between 6 and 15 years. The urine and feces analyzes of 114 school children have identified 62 (54.4%) school children infected. Among schoolchildren examined, 42.1% are infected with schistosomes and soil-transmitted helminths by 28.9% (Table 1). At the baseline, 37.5% of school children were carriers of at least one parasite against 70.1% a year later. The school children infected in the second survey appeared to be significantly ($P < 0.0001$) more numerous than those of the baseline survey, regarding schistosomiasis ($P < 0.0001$). For soil-transmitted helminths difference is not significantly ($P = 0.131$). Considering prevalence of the parasitic species, *Schistosoma haematobium* attained 41.2% as judged by urine analysis, and *Ancylostoma spp.* (27.2%) excreted in the feces. *Trichuris trichiura* (2.6%) and *Schistosoma mansoni* (0.9%) were rarely observed following stool analyses. Based on prevalence, urinary schistosomiasis is the main parasite of Taabo-village.

The intensities of infections reported in Table 2, indicate that whatever the year, the majority of the population is infected with schistosomes i.e more than 75% have a mild infection (<50 eggs in 10 ml of urine for *S. haematobium* and <100 eggs in 1 g of stool for *S. mansoni*) (WHO, 2004). Heavy infections (≥ 50 eggs in 10 ml of urine for *S. haematobium* and ≥ 400 eggs in 1 g of stool for *S. mansoni*) appear to be solely due to *S. haematobium*. As for those who are infected by soil-transmitted helminths, they all have a mild infection (Table 2). It is of note that the intensities of infection of these parasites remained invariant after treatment.

Awareness, prevention and treatment were made by two teachers from the school age population and a community health worker (CHW) to other members of the community. In the general population of Taabo-village, the number of infected individuals is estimated at 70% and yet only 12% were treated between 2008 and 2009 (Table 3). This low rate indicates that there was no enthusiasm in general; however it was more encouraging in schools where 32.9% were treated against 8.2% in the village.

The sociological survey involved 176 people including 78 school-age children and 98 adults. The quantitative information reported in Table 4 indicate that schistosomiasis and soil are considered as diseases by over 65% of respondents. However, the majority states that these parasites do not have serious consequences on their health and more than 95% confirms that they are not dreadful. The concept of illness and fear is determined by a set of characters which are: immobility, pain, costly treatment, lack of effective remedy, contagiousness, disability, lack of knowledge of symptoms and rapid death. To fight against the parasites, the most common practice (19.4%) is the association of pharmaceutical products and plants. In the control project against the diseases in question, the community generally wants to organize neighborhood with awareness as major roles (35.7%) and environmental health (18.4%). According to the qualitative data, people think that these ailments do not require treatment because they are supposed to heal over time. Also they do not know the mode of contamination which they think would be done by drinking dirty water from the lake, spanning the urine of a schistosomiasis patient, or by bathing in the lake water.

	Taabo-village 1		**TOTAL**
	2008	**2009**	
Number of subjects examined	56	58	114
Number of parasitized individuals	21	41	62
Prevalence %	37.5	70.1	54.4
Schistosomiasis			
Number of parasitized individuals	13	35	48
Prevalence (%)	23.2	60.3	42.1
S. haematobium			
Number of parasitized individuals	12	35	47
Prevalence (%)	21.4	60.3	41.2
S. mansoni			
Number of parasitized individuals	1	0	1
Prevalence (%)	1.8	0	0.9
Soil-transmitted helminths			
Number of parasitized individuals	13	20	33
Prevalence (%)	23.2	34.4	28.9
Ancylostoma spp.			
Number of parasitized individuals	13	18	31
Prevalence (%)	23.2	31.0	27.2
T.trichiura			
Number of parasitized individuals	0	3	3
Prevalence (%)	0	5.1	2.6

Table 1. Prevalence of schistosomiasis and soil-transmitted helminths before (2008) and after deworming (2009) in Taabo lake dam in south-center of Côte d'Ivoire

Schistosomiasis		Soil-transmitted helminths Infection intensities (%) in years		
	2008	**2009**	**2008**	**2009**
Light infection	76.9	77.1	100	100
High infection	23.1	22.9	0	0

Table 2. Percentages of intensities of schistosomiasis infection and soil-transmitted helminths in the Taabo lake dam in south-center of Côte d'Ivoire

	Population		
	Workforces	**Treated**	**Treated Percentage**
Attending school	598	197	32.97
Not attending school	3 331	275	8.25
Total	3 929	472	12.01

Table 3. Percentage of treated population to Taabo-village of 2008 – 2009

They use water from Lake dam for all daily activities including laundry, washing dishes, cooking, bathing, swimming and even sometimes for drinking when drinking water is inaccessible. Fishing takes place in the lake, and the water is also used to irrigate nurseries of coffee and cocoa.

	Reactions et reponses to questions	**Workforces**	Percentages
Knowledge of diseases			
Schistosomiasis	Know	128	72.7
	Do not Know	48	27.3
	Serious	39	22.2
	Less serious	137	77.8
soil-transmitted helminths	Know	115	65.3
	Do not Know	61	34.7
	Serious	55	31.2
	Less serious	121	68.8
Communities attitudes	Non dreadful schistosomiasis	168	95.5
	Dreadful schistosomiasis	8	4.5

	Reactions et reponses to questions	Workforces	Percentages
	Non dreadful soil-transmitted helminthes	172	97.7
	Dreadful soil-transmitted helminthes	4	2.3
Practices in communities	None	2	2.1
	Never infected	61	62.2
	Pharmaceutical products	10	10.2
	Medicinal Plants	6	6.1
	Pharmaceutical products + Plants	19	19.4
Control Project	By neighborhood	57	58.1
	Combination	2	2.1
	Gender	9	9.2
	No answer	30	30.6
Role in participation	Decision making	10	10.2
	Environmental health	18	18.4
	Awareness	35	35.7
	Supervision	5	5.1
	No answer	30	30.6

Table 4. Results of sociological surveys conducted in Taabo-village community near the dam Taabo in south-center of Côte d'Ivoire.

4. Discussion

Parasitic diseases highlighted in the locality of the Taabo-village are schistosomiasis and hookworm. Schistosomiasis was the predominant parasitosis. It was followed by ankylostosomiasis. This classification is different from the distribution observed in Africa south of the Sahara where ankytosmosomiasis is top of the list (Hotez et Kamath, 2009). The prevalence of these parasitoses are moderate overall. However, a high prevalence of *Schistosoma haematobium* in the order of 60% was recorded at the end of the study in 2009 where no case of *S. mansoni* infection was observed. The study area is an environment with a high prevalence of urinary schistosomiasis as already reported by N'Goran and colleagues more than 20 years ago (N'Goran et al., 1987).

The high prevalence of 60.3% recorded only a year later, does not demonstrate that reinfection is fast because we have not reviewed all of the students selected in 2008. Rather we made another sample because we adopted a population-based approach to see how the home would evolve in real conditions when the population was aware and had medicines at their disposal. On the contrary, this result reveals that the treatment did not have a great influence on morbidity indicators such as the prevalence and intensity of infection. It is explained by the fact that only 12% of the population was treated. Thus, for the treatments have a significant impact, they must extend at least 75% of the school age population and for a long-term as recommended by the WHO (2012). Based on the categories of prevalences and intensities of infection, we offer an annual treatement of the entire community with praziquantel in the case of schistosomiasis. As for soil-transmitted helminthiasis, albendazole may also be distributed once a year. However, all children of preschool and school age and women of childbearing age and adults at risk should be given priority in accordance with the recommendations of the WHO (WHO, 2004.9; 2010.3). For ongoing management, it would be appropriate after the annual mass distribution campaign to,make anthelmintics available to the public through the channels of teachers and community health worker.

It should be noted that while anthelmintics were made available to the Taabo village's population, very few people were treated. There was no enthusiasm for the treatment for the simple reason that these parasites are considered by the majority of the population as non-serious illnesses and less dreadful. For this population it is not necessary to observe measures of prevention and fight as they think diseases are supposed to heal over time. We think that these perceptions are a major obstacle to control actions by chemotherapy.

To develop an appropriate approach of prevention, we must attract the attention of the population through advocacy and health education as suggested by Monday (Useh, 2012). This awareness action and the population's education aim to significantly alter his perception of the severity of these infections, the effectiveness of existing treatments anthelmintics and the risk behaviors. Emphasis will be placed on the causes of the outbreak of schistosomiasis, the consequences associated with schistosomiasis and soil-transmitted to the modes of transmission of these parasites and the importance of seeking treatment for infections. However, awareness sessions will be done with the involvement of opinion leaders such as religious and customary authorities and groups of associations. Awareness must be held at school in the village, in places of worship and preferably on Sunday, which is the market day or the gathering of this farming population. These control actions will take place between December and February which is the rest period for farmers.

Instead of preventing people from visiting the lake shore, we suggest people to collect water for their domestic activities early in the morning i.e before 10 am or in afternoon after 2:00 p.m. The interval between 10 am and 2 p.m corresponds to the maximum period of cercariae emission in water during which people would better avoid attending it. Moreover, the authorities should ensure that drinking water is accessible and that latrines are available. To reduce transmission, we recommend people not to urinate and defecate in the lake or to defecate far away from the lake.

It must be noted that the relatively low percentage of 23.2% of schistosomiasis, recorded at the beginning of the study has not yet been determined in this locality to our knowledge. This level of prevalence could be explained by the previous effect of control actions. We can mention as examples the mass treatment against schistosomiasis conducted in five primary schools around the dam of Taabo and in hyperendemic primary school of Tiassalé's district that Taabo-village is part of it (N'Goran et al., 1997 and 1998). In addition, control activities are performed in Taabo-village for only about a decade (Esse, 1997; N'Goran et al., 1997, 2001 and 2003). This is also probably the reason why the intensities of infection were mostly minor. Morbidity is less severe in the population examined. Indeed, the population examined would be concerned because it is often affected by the programs against schistosomiasis and soil-transmitted helminthiasis. It could be that the category of population such as adultes that do not fall often in programs against these infections have more severe lesions. This was noted by Keita et al. Mali (Keita et al., 2009).

The prevention and control proposed above should extend at least 75% of the school age population and make long-term as recommended by the WHO (2012). We propose to this end a period of at least five years.

5. Conclusion

The results of this study allow us to identify an approach for prevention and sustainable fight against schistosomiasis and soil-transmitted helminthiasis in the context of a large dam in Côte-d'Ivoire. It is partly based on the awareness of the population in order to change significantly their perception of the seriousness of these infections and the effectiveness of existing anthelmintics treatments. On the other hand, the population will change habits in relation to periods of attendance at the lake and the discharge of excrement in the water. This fight will be the responsibility of community and must be sustained for a long term This community approach of prevention and control proposed at the end of our study is most applicable in the context of eco-epidemiological of large dams, where soil-transmitted helminthiasis and schistosomiasis are generally a serious, but neglected, public health problem.

Acknowledgements

We specially acknowledge the Agence Universitaire de la Francophonie (AUF), which funded the research. The authors wish to thank Mr TP Gonety, Taabo Hospital Director and Dr. L. Adiossan the chief doctor of the said hospital for treatments supervision. We acknowledge inspector of primary teaching, principals and teachers of Taabo-village and the Head of this locality. We also acknowledge the laboratory technicians, KL Lohourignon, M. Traore, S. Diabaté, A.S. Brou, J. Brou, S. Kouadio, M. N'Cho, N. Kouadio and MG Gry for the quality of the work they have done and Mr Zahoui André for the translation from English.

Author details

Nicaise Aya N'Guessan [1], Orsot Niangoran Mathieu[1], Abé N'Doumi Noël[2] and N'Goran Kouakou Eliézer[1]

*Address all correspondence to: nicaisayan@yahoo.fr

1 UFR Biosciences, University of Cocody-Abidjan, Côte d'Ivoire

2 Faculty of Communication Environment and Society, University of Bouaké, Côte d'Ivoire

References

[1] Doumenge JP, Mott KE, Cheung C, Villenave D, Chapuis O, et al. (1987). Atlas of the global distribution of schistosomiasis. World Health Organization, Geneva: 16:398.

[2] Esse AMC. (1997). The impact of hydroelectric dams on the health of local populations: the case of urinary schistosomiasis in the region Taabo. Master's thesis, Science of Man and Society, University of Cocody, Abidjan, Ivory Coast. 30p

[3] Hotez PJ & Kamath A (2009). Neglected tropical diseases in Sub-Sahara Africa: Review of Their prevalence, distribution and disease burden. PLoS Negl Trop Dis, 3, e412.

[4] Katz N, Chaves A, Pellegrino JA (1972). Simple device for quantitative stool thick-smear in Schistosomiasis mansoni. technical. Revista do Instituto Medicina Tropical de São Paulo 14:397-400.

[5] Keita AD, Sacko M, Coulibaly SY, et al. (2009). Imaging of urological tumors in an endemic area of schistosomiasis in Mali. J. Afr. Cancer 1:135-140.

[6] Useh MF (2012). Control of schistosomiasis in Schistosomiasis, In-Tech, ISBN : 978-953-307-852-6. DUI:10.5772/25326

[7] N'Goran EK, Diabaté S, Utzinger J, Sellin B (1997). Changes in human schistosomiasis Levels the after the Construction of Two hydroelectric dams in wide central Ivory Coast. Bull World Health Org 75:541-545.

[8] N'Goran EK, Utzinger J, Gnaka HN, Yapi A, N'Guessan NA, Kigbafori SD et al. (2003). Randomized, double-blind, placebo-controlled trial of oral artemether for the prevention of patent Schistosoma haematobium infections. American Journal of Tropical Medicine and Hygiene 68 (1): 24-32.

[9] N'Goran EK, Utzinger J, N'Guessan NA, Muller I, K Zamble et al. (2001). Reinfection with Schistosoma haematobium following school-based chemotherapy with praziquantel in endemic villages in oven Highly Ivory Coast. Trop Med Int Health 6:817-825.

[10] N'Goran KE, Utzinger J, Traore M, Lengeler C & Tanner M (1998). Rapid identification by questionnaire of the main foci of urinary bilharziasis in central Ivory Coast. Med Trop 58, 253-260. 25.

[11] N'Guessan AN (2003). The fight against schistosomiasis in Côte d'Ivoire : epidemiological factors of complexity and control operational constraints. Thesis, University of Cocody in Abidjan, Ivory Coast.

[12] N'Guessan NA, Acka CA, Utzinger J, N'goran EK (2007). Identification of high risk regions of schistosomiasis in Ivory Coast. Bull Soc Pathol Exot 100(2):119-123.

[13] World Health Organization (2000). Ultrasound in schistosomiasis. A practical guide to the use of ultrasonography standardized for the assessment of schistosomiasis-related morbidity. WHO, document TDR/STR/SCH/00.1

[14] World Health Organization (2001). Schistosoiasis and geohelminthiasis. 19th session of the 54th World health assembly. http://www.who.int/mediacenter/factscheets/fs366/fr/

[15] World Health Organization (2003). Act against worms, Bull PPC, World Health Organization 1: 1-6.

[16] World Health Organization (2004). Act against worms, Bull PPC, World Health Organization 4: 1-10.

[17] World Health Organization (2004a). Fight against helminth infections among school age children. Guide for managers of control programs. World Health Organization, Geneva.

[18] World Health Organization (2004b). Prevention and control of schistosomiasis and soil-transmitted helminthiasis. Report of a WHO expert committee. WHO Technical Report Series N° 912. World Health Organization Geneva.

[19] World Health Organization, UNICEF (2004.9). Schistosomiasis and soil-transmitted helminthiasis: Action of prevention and control of 16/09/2012 (whqlibdoc.who.int/hq/2004/WHO_CDS_CPE_PVC_2004.9_fre.pdf)

[20] World Health Organization (2008a). Act against worms. Bull PPC, World Health Organization 12: 1-8.

[21] World Health Organization, UNICEF (2010.3). Communicable disease epidemiological profile Côte d'Ivoire. (2010.3 whqlibdoc.who.int/hq/2010/WHO_HSE_GAR_DCE_eng.pdf)

[22] World Health Organization (2011). Schistosomiasis. Number of people treated, 2009. Weekly Epidemiological Record 9, 86:73-80.

[23] World Health Organization (2012). Geohelminthiasis. Reminder N°366 of 19/8/2012 http://www.who.int/mediacenter/factscheets/fs366/fr/

[24] Plouvier S, Leroy JC, Colette J (1975). About a simple filtration of urine in the diagnosis of urinary schistosomiasis in mass survey. Med Trop 35:229-230.

[25] Raso G, Matthys B, N'Goran EK, Tanner M, Vounatsou P and Utzinger J (2005). Spatial risk Prediction and mapping of Schistosoma mansoni infections among school children living in western Côte d'Ivoire. Parasitology 131:97-108.

[26] Sellin B and Simonkovich E (1982). Schistosomiasis and dams in Côte d'Ivoire. In : From epidemiology to human geography. Works Tropical and Geographical Papers 48:209-214.

[27] Steinmann P, Keiser J, Bos R, Tanner M, Utzinger J (2006). Schistosomiasis and water resources development: systematic review, meta-analysis, and estimates of people at risk. Infection.thelancet.com 6:411-425.

[28] Utzinger J, N'Goran EK, Ossey YA, Booth M, Traore M et al. (2000). Rapid screening for Schistosoma mansoni in western Côte d'Ivoire using a simple school questionnaire. Bull World Health Org 78 (3):389-397.

Chapter 4

Schistosomiasis

Monday Francis Useh

Additional information is available at the end of the chapter

http://dx.doi.org/10.5772/53553

1. Introduction

Schistosomiasis is a chronic water-borne infection caused by digenetic trematodes that belong to the genus *Schistosoma*. There are two main forms of the disease namely; urinary and intestinal schistosomiasis. The major aetiologic agents of the intestinal form are *Schistosoma mansoni* and *Schistosoma japonicum*. The less common species that have also been associated with intestinal disease are *Schistosoma mekongi, Schistosoma guineensis* and the related species *Schistosoma intercalatum. Schistosoma haematobium* is the only known agent of urogenital schistosomiasis [1]. *S. haematobium* and *S. mansoni* infections have been widely reported in all parts of Nigeria although the former predominates [2].

Schistosomiasis is transmitted by snails. Each of the species is transmitted by a snail of a different species. The intermediate host of *S. haematobium* is a fresh water snail belonging to the genus *Bulinus*. It is a turreted snail with a left-handed opening when looked at with the spire upwards. Three main species are known to harbour the larval stages of schistosomes [3]:

- The Africanus group (sub-genus *Physopsis*) which are involved in the transmission of the disease in eastern, central and west Africa
- The truncatus group (sub-genus *Bulinus)* which transmits infection in the near East and in some parts of Africa and
- The forskalli group. This group has been associated with the transmission of urinary schistosomiasis in Nigeria among other places in Africa.

S. mansoni is transmitted by flattened planorbid snails belonging to the genus *Biomphalaria*. Four main groups have been associated with the transmission of intestinal schistosomiasis in Africa. These include:

- The Pfeifferi group which are the main vectors in Africa
- The sudanica group which occur in both east and west Africa
- The choanomphala which are found in the great lakes and act as agent in Lake Victoria and
- The Alexandrina group which occur sporadically in north, east and south Africa [3]

The intermediate host of *S. japonicum* are operculated snails that belongs to the genus *Oncomelania*. Important species such as *O. hupensis*, *O. nosophora*, *O. formosana* and *O. quadrasi* are involved in the transmission of infection in different areas of Asia where the infection predominates [3].

The role of water bodies in the transmission of infection cannot be over emphasized [4]. Such water bodies include fresh water streams, water accumulated as a consequence of construction of dams and irrigation projects and slow flowing or stagnant water. Although, the main courses of large rivers may not be associated with the transmission of schistosomiasis, but water sustained by them through seasonal flooding and impoundment may provide avenues for the sustenance of the snail intermediate host. Water also provides an opportunity for the cercariae to survive and penetrate the definitive host. Humans are also pivotal in the transmission of schistosomiasis. Through insanitary disposal of urine or faeces, water bodies are contaminated with the eggs of schistosomes. Worldwide, 900 million people do not have access to an improved water source, while an estimated 2.5 billion, half of all people in developing countries lack access to adequate sanitation [5,6]. In rural and poor agricultural communities without pipe-borne water, the locals depend on cercariae infested streams for their economic and recreational needs thereby exposing themselves to infection.

The control of schistosomiasis involves an integrated process directed at the infected subjects, snail intermediate hosts, environmental modification, health education and the provision of pipe-borne water [7]. In this review, the epidemiology, diagnosis and control of schistosomiasis is examined in details with notes on the factors impeding the control of the disease in Africa with inferences drawn from the Nigerian experience.

2. Epidemiology of schistosomiasis

Schistosomiasis is estimated to infect about 240 million people worldwide while an estimated 779 million people (more than 10% of the world population) are at risk of acquiring infection. Although, the transmission of schistosomiasis has been documented in 77 countries worldwide, only 52 of these countries are endemic for the disease, majority of which are in the Africa continent. Forty six [46] of these countries are in Africa. Unlike the situation in Africa, some countries in Latin America and Asia and most countries of the Caribbean and the Middle East have brought down the prevalence of schistosomiasis and prevented severe morbidity from the infection through a concerted public health effort. But in many of these countries, there are still endemic regions and a potential for resurgence exists [8]. About 120 million people infected with schistosomiasis are estimated to be symptomatic while about 20 million develop severe disease. The disability adjusted life years due to schistosomiasis is about 1.7-4.5 million while between 150,000 to 280,000 people are known to die as a consequence of schistosomiasis per year. Africa accounts for 85% of the disease burden [9,10]. Urinay schistosomiasis has been reported in 38 countries in Africa. Annual mortality due to *S. haematobium* infection in east Africa has been estimated at 1 per 1000 infected adults [11]. In Malawi, Save the children's 1998 survey of schoolchildren in Mangochi found that the overall prevalence of schistosomiasis in coastal and upland schools was 36%. In some of the schools, the prevalence was as high as 87% [12]. In a related study in Cameroon, Mba and Useh [13] reported urinary schistosomiasis among 39.2% of the subjects studied. Mixed infection of *S. haematobium* and *S. mansoni* occurred in 4.5% of the subjects. The number of infected subjects treated for the disease using praziquantel rose for 12.4 million in 2006 to 33.5 million in 2010. It is estimated that 90% of those that require treatment live in Africa. This implies that over 60% of people suffering from schistosomiasis particularly in Africa are not able to procure treatment or have access to treatment due to the relatively high cost of praziquantel.

2.1. Schistosomiasis situation in Nigeria

It is estimated that 30 million Nigerians are infected with schistosomiasis. When examined against a projected population of 162 million Nigerians, it becomes clear that over 18.5% of the populace have schistosomiasis. The problem becomes more glaring when the projected population of infected people is examined in terms of those who carry the greatest burden of the disease; in this case, school age children. About 23 years ago, Ejezie *et al* [2] published a major review entitled "the schistosomiasis problem in Nigeria" where they highlighted the embarrassing and increasing endemicity of schistosomiasis without any concrete plan for control. Not much has changed almost two and half decades after. In another landmark review on the "Nigerian environment and parasitic infections", Ejezie [14] noted that "a large proportion of the people consist of men and women who are ignorant of the rules of basic hygiene. These people are entrapped by the worst manifestations of poverty, worsened by infectious tropical diseases, malnutrition, high birth and death rate". They are, as it were, caught in the so-called vicious circle-"they are sick because they are poor, they become poorer because they are sick and sicker because they are poorer" [15]. The problem seems to have grown worst. In the above publication, infection with *S. haematobium* was reported in all the regions in Nigeria with a prevalence as high as 60-75% among schoolchildren in some communities. The endemicity of *S mansoni* was also reported though not as wide spread as the former. Perhaps this report and others encouraged the government of Nigeria to constitute the 'National Schistosomiasis Control Committee". Regrettably, this Committee only existed on paper as funds were not made available to organize operational research to delineate endemic communities for treatment.

The morbidity of schistosomiasis in Nigeria reflects what has been published for endemic countries in Africa and Asia. Infection predominates in schoolchildren aged between 5-19 years and thereby decline following the typical "age verus prevalence/intensity convex curve". An earlier study conducted on urinary schistosomiasis reported a prevalence of 45.4% in Ilorin, Central Nigeria with 25.9% of infected subjects excreting 1,000eggs/10ml urine [16]. In a related study in Adim community located in south south Nigeria, this author and his colleagues reported an overall prevalence of 53.8% with males and females accounting for 53.8% and 53.9% of infection respectively. In this study, the mean haematuria, proteinuria and egg-output were 23.19 ery/ul, 49.9mg/100ml and 37.3 eggs/10ml urine [17]. Three years after, in the absence of a control programme, the prevalence of urinary schistosomiasis in this same community rose astronomically to 90.7% among children out of the school system while those who attended school had a prevalence of 86.8% [18].

The current picture of schistosomiasis endemicity in Nigeria is very worrisome. For instance in their investigation on urinary schistosomiasis around Oyan Reservoir, south west Nigeria, Akinwale *et al* [19] reported a prevalence that ranged from 20.39%-83.9% in some communities around the reservoir. In Bida, north central Nigeria, Banji *et al* [20] reported a prevalence of 28% among school children. Recently, Goselle *et al* [21] reported the endemicity of *S. mansoni* in Jos, north central Nigeria. Yet another study reported on the epidemiology of schistosomiasis in six local government areas in Plateau State, Nigeria [22]. The overall prevalence of infection was 47.8%. Many water bodies in the study communities were colonized by infected *Bulinus* snails. Snail infection rates varied significantly ($P<0.001$) between the dry and wet seasons. Most studies on schistosomiasis are based on the school system. Not much has been done on children out of the school system and on preschool children. In one of such studies among preschool children in a rural community near Abeokuta, south west Nigeria, Ekpo *et al* [23] reported a prevalence of 58.1% with the overall geometric egg count of 1.17 eggs/10ml urine. There is gross lack of work on genital schistosomiasis in Nigeria. With a high prevalence of HIV/AIDS infection in Nigeria, it is important that this be addressed. Genital schistosomiasis particularly in women may have helped to spread the transmission of HIV infection.

2.1.1. Consequences of schistosomiasis infection in Nigeria

The pathology associated with schistosomiasis in Nigeria is consistent with what have been reported in other endemic countries. The pathology of schistosomiasis is essentially a series of chronic inflammatory lesions produced in and around blood vessels by eggs which may be found lodged in practically any viscera or their products and sometimes by dead worms. There are comprehensive studies in the literature on the pathology due to urinary schistosomiasis [24,25,26,27]. In summary disorders such as cercarial dermatitis, haematuria, proteinuria, calcification of bladder, uteric stricture and dilatation, hydronephrosis and squamous cell carcinoma have been reported. Others include multi granulomatas in the bladder and vesicle calculus. Attah [28] noted that the pathology of intestinal schistosomiasis is characterized by the presence of a small superficial ulceration of colonic mucosa, with eggs and granulomas found much more frequently in the serosa than in the mucosa; and by lesions which are secondary to disintegration of eggs and aggravated by oviposition. Hepatic lesions is marked by eosinophilic infiltration of the portal tract with or without eggs. In chronic cases, the major lesion in the liver is 'pipe stem fibrosis', an enlarged liver and fibrosed portal tract with a varying degree of portal vein destruction.

Schistosomal infection has been associated with other negative effects among Nigerian children. These include poor attendance at school, low cognitive ability, educational achievement and malnutrition. This is exemplified in one study in which we treated schoolchildren with urinary schistosomiasis with PZQ and monitor its effect on educational attainment in Adim community of Nigeria. The pass rate among the cohort improved following the first treatment session from 81.4% to 90.7%, latter declined to 84.2% following the second treatment session but the net improvement in performance was statistically significant [29]. On the contrary, Ejezie and Ade-Serrano [30] showed that anthropometric measurements in relation to age, to average marks scored and school attendance were not found to bear any relationship to the intensity of *S. haematobium* infection in Lagos Nigeria. Similarly, Ekanem *et al* [31] did not find any significant impact of infection on anthropometric parameters, school attendance and academic performance among infected children compared to controls in Nigeria. In Kenya, Corbet *et al* [32] showed that intensity of *S mansoni* infection correlated with hepatomegaly, which was more clearly related to nutritional status. Furthermore they noted that children with hepatomegaly were significantly more stunted and/or wasted than those without, and had less variety in their diet. Similarly, Stephenson *et al* [33,34] demonstrated that children infected with *S. haematobium* had evidence of poor nutritional status, with improved growth rates in children and weight gain in undernourished adults following treatment with metrifonate or PZQ. The consequences of infection may be a function of the morbidity of infection in the area, age, nutritional and economic status of the infected subjects.

Educational Performance	**Pre-Treatment N=210**	**Post-treatment 1 N=183**	**Post-treatment 11 N=203**	**X2**	**P**
Total attendance Pupils days	46,902	40,269	40,402		
Attendance rate (%)	86.7	81.5	81.1	2.99	0.22
Days school open	257	270	245		
No passed	171	166	171		
Pass rate	81.4	90.7	84.2	7.2	0.027

Adopted from Meremikwu et al (2000)

Table 1. Effect of treatment on attendance and pass rate in a cohort of school children over three years

3. Diagnosis of schistosomiasis

Diagnosis is pivotal in all aspects of the control of schistosomiasis. Feldmeier *et al* [35] noted that decisions on individual and community treatment, estimations on prognosis and assessment of morbidity, determination of transmission potential, evaluation of treatment and of control measures all build on the results from diagnostic testing. The diagnosis of human schistosomiasis is based on a combination of clinical symptoms, history of residence in an endemic or non-endemic area, parasitological examinations, serological findings and ultrasonography [36]. However all presently available techniques are characterized by diagnostic imperfections or inaccuracies. Consequently, Feldmeier *et al* [35] recommended that selection and application of methods should be related to information being sought while interpretation of test results should take cognizance of the drawbacks and constraints associated with the method being used.

3.1. Clinical diagnosis

The expected clinical conditions include cutaneous lesions, urticaria, eosinophilia and pulmonary disorders. Others include haematuria, cystitis, urinary calculi and vesicular disorders which should be differentiated from other disease conditions giving rise to renal calculi, nephritis, tuberculosis, haemoglobinuria, benign and malignant papillomata. This method of diagnosis is not very sensitive and specific. In endemic areas children may not be able to relay their problem to the physician. On the other hand, primary health care workers who are the first set of health workers to come in contact with infected subjects may not be knowledgeable enough to relate this clinical presentation with schistosomiasis.

3.2. Direct parasitological techniques

Urine egg count is one of the three methods for estimating the intensity of infection; the other two, tissue egg burden and number of worm pairs, can only be determined at autopsy [37]. The WHO [38] noted that quantitative egg count provides reliable baseline data for studies on chemotherapy, malacology, sociology and contamination patterns in defined communities. In the same vein, it also provides information on the transmission potential of different population subgroups. Parasite counts are usually estimated by filtration with nytrel, standard filter paper (Whatman) or by centrifugation of urine. The filtration technique which gives excellent results is applicable in the field [39]. In Africa, filtration with Whatman filter paper is predominantly used in the field and has been associated with reliable and consistent results [17,40]. Smith *et al* [41] reported that in the active stage urinary excretion can be used as an indirect estimate of tissue egg burden and severity of the disease and is particularly relevant for epidemiological studies. In the inactive stage of infection, few or no eggs may be present. Urine egg counts are of limited essence in estimating the prevalence of severe disease in inactive stage of schistosomal disease or in older population. In a related study, a significant correlation was found between haematuria, proteinuria, leucocyturia and intensity of infection as measured by egg excretion in urine [42]. The best correlation between the reagent strip findings and the intensity of infection was obtained when the three parameters were combined. After treatment with metrifonate, the reduction of egg excretion was paralleled by the normalization of the reagent strip findings. Analysis of day-to-day variation demonstrated a similar low variation of the filtration technique and the reagent strip findings. The authors concluded that polyvalent reagent strips may be a useful tool for diagnosis of heavily infected patients under field conditions, as they permit rapid and easy identification of subjects with high egg counts.

Unlike the eggs of *S. haematobium*, the eggs of *S. mansoni*, *S. japonicum* and *S. intercataltum* are passed in faeces. The formol ether concentration technique may be used to demonstrate the spined eggs of any of these parasites. The problem associated with the technique is that it is not field application. Apart from the requirements of a centrifuge and a microscope, the use of ether which is highly flammable poses a hazard. The Kato thick smear technique is more widely used in field work in Africa. The samples can be prepared in the field while examination may be done later.

For community-based studies, enormous human and financial resources are expended to establish those infected before the administration of chemotherapy. A reasonable number of skilled manpower would be required to avoid undue waste of time. In practical terms it is usually not possible to identify infected people the same day and offer them treatment in the field. In some instances during a re-visit for treatment, infected children may miss treatment either because of sickness or lending a helping hand to their parents in the farm. Thus a lot of money that ought to be used to procure treatment is expended on diagnosis. Parasitological confirmation of eggs in urine or stool have been associated with some degree of poor accuracy and sensitivity [43]. The day-to-day variations in excreted egg counts in individual patients [44] and the uneven distribution of eggs in excreta [45] and the occurrence of immature infections [46] are some of the limiting factors. Others include the immune dependence of schistosome egg excretion and the survival of worms after an immunological induced inhibition of fecundity [47]. Nonetheless, the establishment of prevalence and morbidity by the presence of ova is necessary for understanding the epidemiological profile of different endemic foci.

3.3. Detection of pathology and ultrasonography

The introduction of cytoscopy in 1879 [48] facilitated the visualization of bladder pathology as a consequence of *S. haematobium* infection *in vivo*. Pyelographic and histopathological studies have been used to assess urinary tract pathology due to *S. haematobium* infection in Nigeria [24,27,49]. Modern radiological techniques have finally provided a variety of methods for the detection and follow-up of schistosome related morbidity. Such procedures include various radiographic techiques, isotype investigations of the kidney and liver, computed tomography and more recently, ultrasonography [50]. Table 2 is a summary comparing *S. haematobium*-related morbidity with currently available methods of detecting morbidity.

	CYSTOSCOPY	RENAL FUNCTION TEST	X-RAY	COMPUTED TOMOGRAPHY	SONOGRAPHY
A. BLADDER					
Granuloma	+	-	+	+	+
Sandy Patches	+	-	-/+	+	+
Ulcers	+	-	-/+	+	-/+
Cystitis	+	-	-	-/+	-
Stones	+	-	+	+	+
Calcification	-/+	-	+	+	-/+
Polyps	+	-	+	+	+
Carcinoma	+	-	+	+	+
B. URETER					
Hydroureter	-/+	-/+	+	+	-/+
Stricture	-/+	-/+	+	+	-
Dilatation/ Distortion	-	-	+	+	-
Calcification	-/+	-	+	+	-/+
Polyps	-/+	-	+	+	-/+
C. KIDNEY					
Congestion	-	-/+	+	+	+
Hydronephrosis	-	-/+	+	+	+
Performance	-	+	+	+	-

Adopted from Hatz *et al* [50].

Table 2. Comparison reflects possibility of detecting without rating efficiency and applicability.

3.4. Indirect parasitological techniques

3.4.1. Haematuria and proteinuria

The detection of haematuria and proteinuria is widely used in Nigeria and the rest of endemic communities in Africa to diagnose urinary schistosomiasis. Haematuria arises when migrating eggs puncture small capillaries of the viscal plexus to get into the bladder [51]. Haematuria was the first sign to be associated with schistosomiasis [52] while proteinuria was described later. Haematuria is usually seen at the end of urination (terminal haematuria), although haematuria throughout micturition may be seen in some severely infected cases. High levels of urinary protein in *S. haematobium* infection has been linked with nephritis [53], nephritic syndrome [54] and bladder pathology [55]. Some authors have cited the reversibility of proteinuria after treatment to support the renal origin of proteinuria [56,57]. It is now generally accepted that bilharzial proteinuria is of post–renal origin and not a sign of impaired renal function [58].

Several studies have confirmed that the detection of proteinuria and haematuria when used together is a better means to measure morbidity than when used separately [25,40,59]. In Lagos, Nigeria, Ejezie and Ade-Seranno, [40] reported haematuria in 655 of infected children with the greatest intensity in patients with the highest egg output. Relatedly, Mottt *et al* [59] and Tanner *et al* [60] noted that all children between 5-14 years with more than 50 eggs per 10ml of urine had blood in the urine detected by chemical reagent strips. This author and his colleagues tested the usage of the presence/absence of haematuria and proteinuria in monitoring the outcome of treatment of urinary schistosomiasis with artesunate. The mean ova count, haematuria and proteinuria of 87 infected subjects who were treated significantly reduced from 55.5± 1.3ova/10ml urine, 168.6±1.23 ery/μL and 458.6± 1.4 mg/dl to 1.8±0 ova/10ml urine, 9.1±0.4 ery/μL and 65.4 mg/dl respectively ($P<0.05$ in all cases). We therefore concluded that reagent strips are reliable in monitoring the efficacy of treatment with artesunate [61].

Reagent strips are cheap, fast, simple and can be readily integrated into the primary health care programme. But there may be gender bias in females that may lead to under-reporting or over-reporting (false positives). The contamination of urine with menstrual blood would yield false positive results for haematuria. A similar finding may be noted for leucocyturia and proteinuria [62]. The usefulness of a semi-quantitative grading of haematuria as a correlate to intensity of infection has to be questioned in women with schistosomiasis, since the ectopic localization of eggs in the vagina, cervix or the endometrium may lead to contact bleeding, intermenstrual bleeding or to bloody discharge [63]. Evidence for false positive reagent strip readings in women has been shown in a population based study on Pemba Island, Tanzania. A higher prevalence of haematuria readings were observed in women of child-bearing age than in males of similar age, although intensity of infection and morbidity as measured by the number of eggs per unit of urine, and as indicated by pathological ultrsonography was significantly less in women than in men [64]. Vester *et al* [65] reported culture-related biases for mass screening with urine analysis strips. About 15% of schistosomiasis-free Sudanese girls and women circumcised either by the "pharaonic" or the "sunna" method constantly or intermittently show mild haematuria and/or leucocyturia. Since female circumcision is practiced not only in Muslim and Coptic societies in the Sudan, but also in more than 40 ethnic groups in Africa and Arabia [66], false positive reagent strip readings are expected to occur where this tradition and schistosomiasis overlap.

3.4.2. *Rapid Assessment Procedure (RAP) using questionnaires*

A greater proportion of money slated for the control of schistosomiasis is usually spent on diagnosis particularly when eggs are to be counted. The fact that schistosomiasis is focal in distribution with millions of infected subjects in endemic communities showing different prevalence and morbidity rates compound the problem. The problem is more felt in Africa with her lean financial resources but with the largest burden of the disease. The rapid assessment procedure was conceived to maximize resources in diagnosis which could be directed to possible chemotherapeutic control of infection

The RAP involves the use of a rapid and inexpensive method to identify communities with a high prevalence of and morbidity due to urinary schistosomiasis. It is based on using simple questionnaires to find out how frequent schistosomiasis is in a community [67]. Kroeger [68] and Ross and Vaughan [69] showed that health interview surveys can be used in both developed and developing countries to assess morbidity as it is perceived by community members, and to investigate the utilization patterns of health services. Tanner [70] demonstrated that asking the beneficiaries of the health system about their perceptions of disease and health problems, and especially about their priorities with regard to health related actions, can add an important element in the health planning cycle. Lengeler *et al* [71] observed that indirect health interview represents a methodical evolution of the traditional interview approach by the fact that questionnaires are not administered directly by the investigators or their field staff to the key informants. Rather, they are distributed through an existing administrative channel and self-administered by the recipients. The school system is therefore the appropriate structure to base a study on the prevalence of schistosomiasis. This is anchored on the fact that those who bear the greatest burden of the disease can be easily reached through this channel. Additionally, schools are widely cited and are very likely to be located in remote endemic areas. Thirdly, teachers are competent enough with minimal training to carry out an exercise of this nature.

Several epidemiological studies are available in the literature that tested the usefulness of this mode of diagnosis. Useh and Ejezie [72] worked on the "evaluation and validation of the questionnaire approach for the diagnosis of urinary schistosomiasis in Biase Local Government Area of Nigeria among school pupils". The questionnaire which enquired whether pupils had urinary schistosomiasis or blood in urine in the preceding month, was administered by class teachers to the pupils. Urines samples collected for the validation of the questionnaire diagnosis was also examined using dipsticks (by teachers and the research team). There was a strong positive correlation between the pupils's knowledge of schistosomiasis as a disease and the reported presence of blood in urine (r=0.96) although the later was a better indicator of the disease. The questionnaire technique (blood in urine) gave a comparable sensitivity (85.8%), specificity (81.4%), positive and negative predictive values (96.6% and 47.9%) to the dipstick test with values of 96.6%, 88.4%, 98% and 69.1% respectively. Teachers were able to detect haematuria with a high degree of accuracy. We found this approach to be simple, cost-effective and reliable and recommended its usage in other endemic settings with large land mass and dense population like Nigeria (See Table 3).

Survey Method	TP a	FP B	FN C	TN d	SENS (%)	SPEC (%)	PPV (%)	NPV (%)	VAL (%)	BIAS (%)	P Value
Blood in Urine	229	9	38	35	85.8	81.4	96.6	47.9	83.3	88.8	P<0.001
Schistosomiasis	207	15	60	28	77.5	65.1	93.2	31.8	73.4	83.1	P<0.001
TDST	231	7	36	36	86.5	83.7	97.1	50.0	84.3	89.1	P<0.001
RDST	250	5	17	38	93.6	88.4	98.0	69.1	91.9	95.5	P<0.001

True Positives, TP were defined as those with ova in urine (n=267). Altogether 310 pupils were examined.

TN- True Negative, FP- False Positive, FN- False Negative

SENS- Sensitivity, SPEC – Specificity, PPV- Positive Predictive Value, NPV- Negative Predictive Value, TDST- Teachers Dipstick Testing, RDST- Researchers Dipstick Testing.

Adopted from Useh and Ejezie, [72].

Table 3. Comparison of the performance of different survey methods in relation to parasitologically confirmed diagnosis

Elsewhere, self-administered questionnaires, distributed by existing administrative channels to village party chairmen, head teachers and school children, showed good diagnostic performance for the qualitative assessment of urinary schistosomisasis endemicity. At a cost 34 times below that of the WHO-recommended parasitological screening strategy, the school children's questionnaire allowed the screening of 75 out of 77 schools of a rural Tanzanian district in 6 weeks, and the exclusion of schools not at high risk for urinary schistosomiasis with over 90% confidence. The head teacher and party chairmen questionnaires made it possible to assess the perceived importance of a spectrum of diseases and symptoms, among which was schistosomiasis. The priority rank of schistosomiasis control was strongly correlated with the prevalence rate of the disease in the community. The questionnaires also looked at the prioritization of health among other community issues and thus contributed important information for planning at the district level [73].

Using questionnaires facilitate immense savings in cost as well as reaching a vast land mass. However, in areas of low school attendance, reliable information may not be collected. Infected but unidentified school-age children that are out of school would invalidate control efforts, as they would continuously contaminate water bodies. Other limitations as outlined by Chitsulo *et al* [67] are-

- results obtained with school children may not always be typical for the whole community especially if a lot of the children of this age are not in school or where one sex is badly under-represented
- the methodology does not identify which child is infected. To obtain this information, a second step using conventional diagnostic method would be necessary
- true prevalence is usually underestimated since the method relies on re-call as those who are mildly infected may not recall having had haematuria
- in some countries, girls and boys may perceive the disease differently or give different answers to questions asked about it.

3.5. Immunodiagnosis

Immunodiagnositic methods are so far the only alternative to parasitological test. They allow the demonstration of specific anti-schistosomal antibodies and to a certain extent, the tracing of circulating antigens and/or immune complexes in sera of parasite carriers [36]. Wilkins *et al* [55] noted that they offer the most practical assays for epidemiological studies and patient management. They are particularly valuable if the density of the parasites (or their developmental stages) in a specimen is very low or if the biology of the parasite does not allow its direct demonstration e.g localization of certain stages in internal organs.

Serological procedures such as immunodiffusion, complement fixation test, indirect haemagglutination assay, immunoflourescent antibody assay have been used for the diagnosis of schistosomiasis. Others include enzyme linked immunosorbent (ELISA), radioimmunoassy and radio-allegrosorbent assay among others. The relevance of antibody detection in the diagnosis of schistosomiasis has been reviewed in great details by Hamilton *et al* [74]. They concluded that due to the relative insensitivity of both parasitology and antigen detection, antibody detection methods could find increasing use in situations of low infection intensity. The performance of antibody detection for the diagnosis of schistosomiasis has been tested in Kenya. Approximately 1500 blood samples from 3 areas with endemic schistosomiasis and from a non-endemic control area, were tested for their antibody reactivity in ELISA. The results were compared with infection status determined by parasitological examination. Two test antigens were used ;unfractionated *S. mansoni* egg homogenate (SEA) and CEF6, a partially purified fraction of SEA containing 2 cationic antigens. Blood from patients with *S. haematobium* infection cross-reacted significantly with the two *S. mansoni* antigen preparations, but reactivity against CEF6 appeared more specifically indicative of *S. mansoni* infection. There was a significant positive correlation between blood ELISA results and the number of eggs excreted by infected subjects in the area endemic for *S. mansoni* only. Highest correlation coefficients were obtained in children aged 10 years and CEF6 gave marginally higher correlation coefficient than SEA. The graphs of prevalence and intensity of schistosome infection drawn from the serological results were similar in shape to the graph of these 2 quantities based on parasitological results, and the results indicate that serology merits wider use as an epidemiological tool for determining infection status in schistosomiasis [75]. In a different but related study, the relative concentration of IgM and IgG antibodies to *S. mansoni* soluble egg antigen were evaluated in paired samples of venous blood, sera and buffer elutes of capillary blood drops dried on filter papers [76]. The samples were obtained from school children at early and chronic stages of schistosomiasis diagnosed on the basis of history, clinical symptomatology and parasitological criteria. ELISA simultaneously performed, revealed paired samples to display comparable antibody levels in all cases. Samples from children with early schistosomiasis had specific IgM : IgG ratios greater than 1 in sera and blood elutes. This ratio, however was less than 1 in samples from chronically infected children. The specific advantages of this simplified technique are the use of anti-SEA antibodies in finger-stick blood elutes, rather than sera or venous blood to serologically diagnose schistosomiasis and to differentiate early from chronic infections particularly when used for mass screening such as epidemiological surveys. Elsewhere, Mclaren *et al* [77] showed that *S. mansoni* SEA gave a sensitivity of 92.3% in diagnosing *S. haematobium* infection and 96.2% for *S. mansoni* and a specificity of 97.4% in ELISA. Recently, Chand *et al* [78] reported on the development of a new assay for the diagnosis of schistosomiasis, using cercarial antigens. They showed that the cercarial antigen assay was equivalent to the SEA assay for serodiagnosis of schistosomiasis in a non-endemic setting. Since the cercarial antigens is more easily obtained and prepared than SEA, the authors inferred this assay may be preferred for routine clinical use and may be amenable for scaling up.

Although the application of serological tests has, without doubt, contributed to epidemiological surveys, such studies are of limited use because some of the tests lack reasonable levels of acceptable sensitivity and specificity or are technically difficult to be carried out in field surveys. Other drawbacks as outlined by Weiland [36] are;

- inability to indicate the intensity of infection or differentiate active from chronic infection
- no correlation between morbidity and sero-reactivity

- cross-reaction with antibodies to other helminthes including animal schistosomes
- unresolved seropositivity remain for years after treatment or after an infection has died out.

The greatest impediment hindering the utilization of immunodiagnosis in third world countries particularly in Africa is lack of financial resources to procure the sophisticated equipment required to carry out some of these procedures and the training of skilled manpower to handle them.

3.6. Rapid diagnostic test

The advent of rapid diagnostic tests has facilitated the immediate treatment of subjects with infectious diseases in the field after diagnosis. Results are usually available within 30 minutes compared to the conventional tests. Apart from its simplicity and ease of carrying out devoid of technicality, the availability of electricity is not required. Rapid diagnostic tests are being deployed in endemic countries for the identification of subjects with malaria, HIV and hepatitis for prompt treatment. Encouraging reports are available in the literature on the development of rapid diagnostic test for schistosomiasis. De jonge *et al* [79] developed a reagent strip test for detection of circulating cathodic antigen in urine. In a related study, Bosompem *et al* [80] showed that *S. haematobium* antigen complexed with complement C3 can be isolated from the urine of infected persons by using a mouse monoclonal antibody. These investigators demonstrated that goat anti-human C3 would also detect schistosome antigen/complement complex in urine of infected persons used as case-controls and subsequently developed a monoclonal antibody dipstick test on the basis of these findings. However, a lot of standardization would be required before these strips are approved by the WHO and other regulatory organizations for deployment in endemic countries.

4. Control of schistosomiasis

The cardinal objective in the control of schistosomiasis is the reduction of morbidity and mortality to levels below public health significance. Over the years, emphasis has shifted from the non-realizable goal of eradication to the more realistic goal of morbidity control. In this context, Gemmel *et al* [81], defined "a control programme" as the "implementation of specific measures by a disease control authority to limit the incidence of the disease". Such implementation may involve specific technical interventions and perhaps legislation to enforce compliance. The success of this type of approach is predicated on an accurate ecological diagnosis, that is, a diagnosis of the human community, its parasitological characteristics, its physico-geographical environmental attributes and man's behavioural attitudes and customs [82].

The enormous morbidity associated with schistosomiasis which ranks it next to malaria in terms of public health significance re-emphasizes the need for a coordinated and sustainable means for the control of the disease. There is a consensus of opinion that the control of the disease should be integrated. In this model of control, King [83] identified the applicable approaches as:

- Population based chemotherapy
- Snail control which involves habitat modification and use of plant and chemical molluscicides,
- Proper treatment of sewage,
- Good environmental engineering designs for the development of irrigation and hydroelectric schemes to limit the availability of breeding grounds for the snail vectors
- Provision of clean and safe piped water and
- Massive health education and mobilization of the population to claim ownership of the programme

The WHO Expert Committee on Epidemiology and Control of Schistosomiasis took a holistic approach at the control of the disease and noted that "comprehensive understanding of the environment, demographic, social, human behavioural and economic factors" in schistosomiasis is essential for the design of control programmes that are successful in the long run [84]. With the advent of praziquantel (PZQ) as a safe and efficacious drug for the treatment of schistosomiasis, the WHO in 1991 reinforced its 1984 recommendation to shift from transmission control (focusing on the prevalence of infection) to morbidity control (laying emphasis on intensity of infection) [8]. Morbidity control will not only reduce the number of people infected but it will also drastically reduce environmental contamination with the eggs even when cure is not attained. A drastic reduction of the pollution of the environment with the eggs would also reduce the chances of transmission. Should this occur at a level below public health importance, the probability of eventual elimination of disease is certain with a sustained integrated approach

4.1. Chemotherapeutic control of schistosomiasis

Of all the methods of control listed above, chemotherapy is the only one that is widely used presently in endemic areas for the control of morbidity due to schistosomiasis. Among the first group of drugs used for the treatment of schistosomiasis included; antimonials, niridazole, hycanthone, lucanthone, oxamniquine and albendazole. PZQ is currently used for the treatment of all the species while metrifonate is active against *S. haematobium* only. Recently, artemisinins earlier synthesized for the treatment of malaria infection is being used in some endemic communities to treat schistosomiasis. The WHO [11] identified four approaches in the administration of chemotherapy programme namely;

i. Mass treatment: treatment of the entire population. This is often limited by availability of finance.

ii. Selective population treatment: treatment of infected persons identified by a diagnostic survey of the whole population

iii. Selective group treatment: treatment of all or infected members of a high risk age or occupational group

iv. Phased treatment: use of the above strategies in a sequence of progressively greater selectivity.

Only the chemotherapeutic form of control of schistosomiasis is covered in the present review. This does not in any way reduce the importance of the other methods. It has already been emphasized above that the sustainable control of schistosomiasis involves the integration of several methods listed above. A comprehensive review on the control of schistosomiasis by this author can be found elsewhere [85]. In the next few paragraphs, the modes of action of several drugs use for the treatment of schistosomiasis are examined.

4.1.1. Praziquantel (PZQ)

4.1.1.1. Biochemical properties and pharmacokinetics

Praziquantel (PZO) is the drug of choice for the treatment of schistosomiasis. It is a broad spectrum anti-schistosomal which is principally active against the adult stage of all the schistosome species infective to man. It is a 2-cyclohexycarbonyl 1,2,3,6,7,11b-hexahydro-4H-pyrazino(2,1-a Isoquinolin-4one) compound with a melting point at 136-140C. It was developed in the laboratories for Parasitological Research of Bayer AG and Merck KGaA in Germany (Elbert and Darmstadt) in the mid 1970s. It has a molecular mass of 312.411 with a serum half life of 0.8 to 1.5 hours in adults with normal liver and kidney function and is mainly excreted in urine. PZQ is a white crystalline powder with bitter taste. It is stable under normal storage conditions. Although, it is insoluble in water, it is soluble in chloroform, dimethylsulfoxide and ethanol. It is sold as a racemate mixture consisting of equal parts of 'laevo' and 'dextro' isomers, of which only the laevo component displays anti-schistosomal properties.

The recommended dose of PZO is 40 mg/kg body weight. The drug is available as a 600mg tablet. The quality of PZQ (proprietary and generic) currently available in the market is quite high and acceptable. Thirty four [34] PZQ samples from different manufacturers were collected at the user level in various countries and subjected to quantitative analysis of active ingredient, purity, disintegration and dissolution in accordance with established pharmacopoeial standards. The results showed that most of the samples were of high quality except two samples from the same manufacturer that had no PZQ [86]. About 90% of the damage done to organ function is known to reverse six months following the administration of PZQ. Although it is exceptionally well tolerated, reported side –effects include abdominal discomfort, nausea, headache, dizziness, drowsiness and pyrexia especially in subjects with high egg counts [87].

4.1.1.2. Mode of action of PZO

The mode of action of PZQ has been extensively reviewed elsewhere [88,89]. The exact mechanisms of action of PZQ is still poorly understood. PZQ is known to induce rapid calcium influx that distort the morhoplogy and physiology of schistosome. Jeziorski and Greenberg [90] showed that the B subunits of voltage-gated Ca^{2+} channels is the prime molecular target of PZQ. It has recently been reported that cytochalasin D abolished the schistosomicicidal activity of PZQ but calcium influx into PZQ exposed schistosomes was not halted. This therefore raises doubts whether calcium influx is essential in the antischistosomal activity of

PZQ [91]. PZQ induces contraction of schistosomes which manifest in paralysis in the contracted state. Additionally, vacuolation and blebbing near and on the surface of the worm have equally been reported [92].

PZQ is known to increase exposure of antigens on the worm surface. It is believed that this in turn renders the worm more susceptible to antibody attack. Doenhoff *et al* [93] inferred that this drug induced antigen exposure is assumed to account for the synergistic effect between PZQ and the host antibodies in killing worms invivo. Recently, it has been shown that PZQ seems to interfere with adenosine uptake in cultured worms. This may have therapeutical relevance given that the schistosome is unable to synthesize purines such as adenosine *de novo*. It may be assumed that the drug interferes with schistosome's obligate need to acquire adenosine from its host. This is confounding as a relationship between Ca^{2+} channels and adenosine receptors has been demonstrated in cells of some other animals and adenosine can antagonize Ca^{2+} release. This informs the inference drawn by Angelucci *et al* [94] that PZQ-induced Ca^{2+} influx and adenosine receptor blockade may be connected.

4.1.1.3. Oxamniquine – Molecular structure and pharmacokinetics

Oxamniquine was first described in the late 1960s. The compound is 6-hydromethyl-2-isopropyl-aminomethyl-7-nitro 1,2,4-tetrahydroquinoline. It is produced by biological processes. The drug is administered as 15mg/kg body weight for adults while children are treated with 20mg/kg given in two doses of 10mg/kg each in an interval of 3-8 hours. It is extensively metabolised through oxidation process. The metabolites are active and excreted in urine. The side effects are mild, transient and well tolerated especially when given after a meal [95].

4.1.1.4. Mode of action

Unlike PZQ, the mechanism of action of oxamniquine is fairly well understood. Oxamniquine is only active against *S. mansoni* but not effective against *S. haematobium* and *S. japonicum*. The active ingredient is tetrahydroquinoline which acts on the adult *S. mansoni* and immature invasive stages, with males more susceptible than the females. Its anticholinergic effect, which increases parasite motility and inhibits nucleic acid synthesis, has no notable effect on the other *Schistosome* species [96]. The mechanism of action of oxamniquine is related to irreversible inhibition of nucleic acid metabolism of the parasite. The drug is activated in a single step, in which the *Schistosoma* enzyme converts the oxamniquine to an ester, and spontaneously dissociates resulting in an electrophilic reactant and alkylation of the Schistosoma DNA. Worm death is associated with the formation of sub-tegumental vesicules in adult parasites. Different responses are observed after therapy, with less specific morphological alteration and hepatic shifts, occurring over a period of six days post treatment [95].

4.1.1.5. Metrifonate

Metrifonate was initially introduced as an insecticide in 1952, but later in 1960, it was used to treat helminth infection. The drug also refer to as trichlorophone is a organophosphorus ester which is only active against *S.haematobium*. It is rapidly absorbed, metabolized and excreted. The metabolic pathway yields DDVP (2,2-dichlorovinyl dimethylphosphate), a cholin esterase inhibitor which is the active compound. The mechanism of action is not known. It is relatively cheap and is not toxic. Metrifonate is administered as 7.5-10 mg/kg body weight, given in three divided doses in two weeks interval. Among the side effects reported following the administration of the drug include abdominal pains, diarrhoea, fatigue and muscular weakness which dissipates within 12 -24 hours [97]. The reasoning behind the widely spread dosage has to do with its inhibitory effects on red cells and plasma cholinesterase.

Metrifonate is not currently used for the treatment of urinary schistosomiasis. Several reasons account for this. One of which is poor compliance by patients as a result of the spacing and multiple dosing. The second reason is reduced level of efficacy. For instance, Mgeni *et al* [98] reported a cure rate of 40% and egg reduction rate of 90% in Zanzibar. Lastly, the advent of PZQ with its superior efficacy rate and broad spectrum activity meant that it was no longer cost effective and sustainable to rely on metrifonate.

4.1.1.6. Artemisinin and its derivatives – Biochemical characteristics and pharmacokinetics

The artemisinins though syntheised for the treatment of malaria is the newest drug used for the treatment of schistosomiasis. Unlike PZQ, which is active against the adult stages of the parasite, artemisinin is active against the immature stage of parasite. It is a sequitterpene lactone with a peroxide group, obtained from the leaves of the plant, *Artemisia annua* which are grown in Central Europe, China, USA and Argentina among others. The major derivatives of artemisinin are artesunate, artemether, arteether with dihydroartemisinin as the principal active metabolite. Primarily they are antimalarials, but the anti-schistosomal properties were discovered by Chinese scientists in the 1980s especially for the treatment of *S japonicum* infection [99]. They are well tolerated with only minor side effects.

4.1.1.7. Mode of action of artemisinin

The precise mode of action of this drug is not known. Artemether is the most potent. It exhibits the highest level of activity on one to three weeks old liver stages of the parasite. When a dosage of 6mg/kg weight is administered, it kills the schistosomulas during the first 21 days. The invasive and adult stages are less affected and the adult females are more susceptible than the males [100]. Following treatment, artemether induces severe and extensive tegumental damage and significant reduction in glycogen contents through the inhibition of glycolsis, but the onset of this alteration is slow. It also hinders the development of egg laying adult worm pairs [101].

PZQ is currently the drug of choice for the treatment of all forms of the disease. It is safe and well tolerated. Readers are referred to a very detailed review on "praziquantel: its use in control of control of schistosomiasis in sub-Saharan Africa and current research needs [89] and "praziquantel: mechanisms of action, resistance and new derivatives for schistosomiasis" [88]. Elsewhere, we reported on the high efficacy and tolerability of PZQ [102] and artesunate [103] for the treatment of urinary schistosomiasis in Nigeria.These authors noted that despite the fact that PZQ is being widely used, there is no clinically relevant evidence for resistance to date, but worrying low-cure rates have been recorded in some studies. They also observed that there is also no assurance that PZQ and/or Schistosomes are in any way unique and that resistant organisms will not be selected as a result of widespread usage. Artesiminis and the related 1,2,4-trioxolanes are now promising antischistosomal compounds, as are inhibitors of a schistosome-specific bifunctional enzyme, thioredoxin-glutathione reductase. In some endemic communities, artesunate is also used for the treatment of malaria singly or in combination. Therefore, where artesunate is used for the treatment of urinary schistosomiasis, resistance may likely develop to malaria. It is pertinent to do an analysis on why schistosomiasis is still highly endemic in some parts of Africa including Nigeria when a potent drug is available for the management of the disorder.

4.1.1.8. Impediments of control of schistosomiais

Several factors are responsible for the continuing endemicity of schistosomiasis in Africa. Some of the factors are examined below;

4.1.1.8.1. High cost of PZQ

Richards [104] identified community-based annual mass drug administration with safe and effective oral drugs as the principal strategy for the control of onchocerciasis, lymphatic filariasis and schistosomiasis. It has been demonstrated that annual treatments with the microfilaricide ivermectin (Mectizan, donated by Merck &Co., Inc.) prevents severe eye disease and skin manifestations of onchocerciasis while the transmission of LF by mosquitoes can be interrupted in Africa by annual single-dose combination therapy with ivermectin and albendazole (donated by GlaxoSmithKline) [105]. Mass distribution of PZQ can significantly reduce schistosomiasis morbidity [106]. However, unlike ivermectin and albendazole, PZQ is not donated and costs approximately US $0.20. Schistosomiasis is a disease that affects poor rural agricultural workers who in most cases cannot afford the cost of PZQ. This is one of the greatest impediments in the control of the disease.

4.1.1.8.2. Lack of political commitment and provision of finance

Until recently, there was no sustained political and financial commitment by the WHO and her health-related agencies and governments of schistosomiasis endemic countries towards the control of schistosomiasis. The success story reported in the control of schistosomiasis in Brazil, China, Egypt, Laos and the Philippines [10,107,108] is an encouragement that the disease can be controlled when the right programmes and processes are in place. Over the years, emphasis on funding of infectious disease control was placed on HIV/AIDS, malaria and tuberculosis/leprosy. That informed the categorization of schistosomiasis as one of the neglected tropical diseases. However, the situation changed during the 54th World Health Assembly held in May, 2001 where resolution WHA 54.19 namely that at least 75% of school-age children in the high-burden regions should be treated regularly with PZQ. This was further enhanced by the launch of the Schistosomiasis Control Initiative [SCI] supported by a US$ 30 million grant from the Bill and Melina Gates Foundation. The SCI is a partnership between Imperial College, London, UK; the Seattle-based Gates Foundation, WHO, Geneva; Harvard School of Public Health, Boston and high-burden country representatives. This renewed interest has encouraged the Carter Centre to be involved in the control of schistosomiasis in Nigeria. The Centre is assisting in the control of schistosomiasis in three states namely; Plateau, Nasarawa and Delta. The Centre is doing this by using the grassroots distribution system of health workers and village volunteers for onchocerciasis to also deliver health education and conduct mass drug administration with PZQ annually in areas affected by both parasites. Since 1999, this programme has delivered a cumulative total of 1,079,335 treatments with PZQ. Studies in a sample of villages in two areas showed a reduction in prevalence of bloody urine assessed by dipsticks from 47% in 1999 to 8% in 2002, after just two years of annual treatments [109]. This success means that LF, onchoceriasis and schistosomiasis can be treated by community health workers at the same time thereby saving enormous cost as a recent clinical trial in Thailand found no clinically relevant pharmacokinetic changes or adverse reactions when ivermectin, PZQ and albendazole were given concurrently [110]

4.1.1.8.3. Lack of strong health system

The health system of many countries in the developing world are not synchronized and integrated. This renders the delivery of health packages difficult and cumbersome. However, there is a conseneus that strong, well integrated and effective health systems are essentials to reduce disease burden and to achieving the health related MDGs. A Strong health systems typically consist of seven building blocks [111,112]. These include: service delivery, governance structures, financial mechanisms, human resources, medicines and technology supply system, health information system and participatory community mechanisms (people). In an ideal situation, these seven components must exist and work together to generate quality (accessible, equitable, responsive health care)

4.1.1.8.4. Health failures

Failures associated with the planning and delivery of healthcare are critical issues that should be targeted to ensure success in the control of infectious diseases including schistosoimasis. In this context, Mahoney and Morel [113] argued that innovation disparity has created 3 kinds of "health failures" namely "science failure, market failure and public health failure". Science failure refers "to a lack of knowledge and tools to address health problems e.g there are still no effective vaccines or drugs for schistosomiasis". Market failures happen "when stock-outs occur due to high demand or when the purchase costs of drugs, vaccines and health interventions prevent the poor from accessing them". Often the new drugs and diagnostics are very expensive to develop and /or require sophisticated technical and health infrastructure for optimal use. Public health failure arises "due to lack of good governance, transparency and effective delivery systems and a clear articulation of priorities and values". Political and economic instability, cultural and religious barriers and shift in government priorities can block the uptake and implementation of health innovations. This is particularly true in Africa where frequent changes of government and dislocation of communities as a result of natural disasters and inter and intra-tribal wars have contributed to hinder outcome of disease control programmes.

5. Development of a schistosome vaccine

Despite the existence of effective chemotherapeutic agents, progress towards controlling schistosomiasis has been slow. Additionally, the possible development of resistance to PZQ and other compounds, rapid re-infection and the overall economic cost, demand that other approaches be pursued [114]. Butterworth *et al* [115] argued that the aim of vaccination is to reduce morbidity. As in the various animal models, immunity in humans appears to be frequently incomplete. "Immune" adults often do become infected, but at lower intensities than "susceptible" children. Several investigations have confirmed that the severity of clinical disease is dependent on intensity of infection rather than simply the presence or absence of infection [116,117] implying that even an incomplete immunity may be of considerable value.

An excellent review on the search for a schistosome vaccine was published not too long ago [118]. These authors rightly chronicled the search for the discovery of candidate vaccine molecules to have transited through mining crude extracts, monoclonal antibody targets, anti-idiotypes, expression library screening and immunogenicity. The early disappointment that was recorded with the vaccination of mice with crude worm extracts or purified components, followed by cercarial challenge [119,120] and utilizing the idea of concomitant immunity [121] were equally reviewed. Wilson and Coulson [118] concluded that the sequencing of *S. mansoni* transriptome and genome and the development of proteomic and microarray technologies has drastically improved the possibilities for identiflying novel vaccine candidates, particularly proteins secreted from or exposed at the surface of schistosomula and adult worms. The parameters of an attenuated schistosome vaccine has been evaluated in the Olive Baboon [122]. Five exposures of baboons to the attenuated schistosome vaccine gave greater protection than three exposures, but this attenuation was not sustained when challenge was delayed. Within the scope of the data collected, faecal and circulating antigen levels did not accurately predict the observed worm burdens. Levels of immunoglobulin G at challenge correlated best with protection, but there was little evidence of a recall response. In a related study in baboons, Coulson and Kariuki [123] showed that neither a preceding infection, terminated by chemotherapy, nor an ongoing chronic infection affected the level of protection. Whilst IgM responses to vaccination or infection were short-lived, IgG responses rose with each successive exposure to vaccine.

The greatest hope for the discovery of a schistosome vaccine lies in Sh28GST which has already undergone Phases 1 and 2 human trials [124]. No adverse side effects were recorded in human recipients and high titres of antibodies were elicited in Phase 1 and phase 2 trials [125]. The results of phase 3 human trials is being awaited. As noted by Curwen *et al* [126] and Dillion *et al* [127], current advances in post-genomic techniques are providing new avenues and hope to identify the secreted and surface-exposed antigens that mediate protection. The search must be sustained as vaccination is the most cost-effective and sustainable means of controlling endemic infectious diseases.

6. Conclusion

Schistosomiasis is still endemic in many parts of Africa particularly Nigeria. Activities related to electric power development/generation and agriculture have extended areas of endemicity just as new foci of infection are being described. The control of schistosomiasis requires an integrated process. However, chemotherapy with PZQ is the mainstay for the control of the disease in the short-term. Poverty on the part of infected subjects, lack of deployment of political and financial resources by disease endemic countries are the major factors limiting the control of the disease. The global economic recession has contributed in reducing financial resources available through bilateral and multilateral avenues for the control of the infectious diseases just as increase in international travels and tourism have led to the reporting of "imported schistosomiasis" in non-endemic countries.

Recommendation

The following recommendations are suggested for the control of schistosomiasis;

- Governments of disease endemic countries should show serious political and financial commitment towards the control of schistosomiasis. Overall, the health sector should be funded in line with the recommendation of the WHO.
- Pharmaceutical companies should be encourage to donate PZQ free as is obtainable with albendazole and ivermectin or in the alternative reduce the cost of the drug.
- The delivery of PZQ should be integrated into ongoing programme of distribution of ivermectin and albendazole by community health workers as it has been shown that taking the three drugs concurrently is safe and effective
- There should be a deliberate policy of providing piped water in endemic communities to reduce the chances of coming in contact with cercariae infested water bodies
- Researchers should be encouraged to develop rapid diagnostic and cost-effective test based on antibody detection which can provide results within 15-20 minutes in the field for the diagnosis of schistomiasis and instant treatment.
- More researches are required to hasten the development of a vaccine for schistosomiasis. This is the only means of long term control of this disease.

Acknowledgments

I wish to appreciate the assistance rendered by my wife; Mary and my daughter; Etini during the preparation of this manuscript. I am indebted to all the colleagues whose references are listed below which have greatly enhance the quality of the manuscript.

Author details

Monday Francis Useh

University of Calabar, Calabar, Nigeria

References

[1] World Health Organization(2012). Fact sheet on schistosomiasis, WHO, Geneva.

[2] Ejezie, G. C., Gemade, E. I. I. &Utsalo, S. J. (1989). The schistosomiasis problem in Nigeria. *Journal of Hygiene Epidemiology, Microbiology & Immunology*, 33, 167-79.

[3] Muller, R. (1975). Worms and Diseases: a manual of medical helminthology (1st Edition), Heinemann, London, 7-20.

[4] Useh, M. F. & Ejezie, G. C. (1999). Modification of behaviour and attitude in the control of schistosomiasis. 1. Observations on water-contact patterns and perceptions of infection. *Annals of Tropical Medicine and Parasitology*, 93(7), 711-720.

[5] World Health Organisation/United Nations International Children Emergency Fund Joint Monitoring Programme for water supply and sanitation (2010). Progress on sanitation and drinking water- 2010 update, Geneva, WHO

[6] United Nations Organization (2007). Coping with water scarcity- Challenges of the 21st century. Rome, Food & Agricultural Organization, UN.

[7] Davis, A. (1989). Operation research in schistosomiasis control. *Tropical Medicine and Parasitology*, 40, 125-129.

[8] Bruun, B & Aagaard-Hansen, J. (2008). *The social context of schistosomiasis and its control- An introduction and annotated bibliography*. UNICEF/UNDP/World Bank/WHO, Switzerland, 19-42

[9] Steinmann, P. *et al* (2006). Schistosomiasis and water resources development: systematic review, meta-analysis and estimates of population at risk. *The Lancet Infectious Diseases*, 6(7),411-425.

[10] World Health Organisation (2002). Prevention and control of schistosomiasis and soil-transmitted helmithiasis. Report of a WHO Expert Committee. Geneva, World Health Organisation (WHO Technical Report Series, No 912).

[11] World Health Organisation (1993). The control of schistosomiasis. Second Report of WHO Committee, WHO/TRS/830, 1-26

[12] Bobrow, E. (1999). Child health in learning and development settings. A baseline report for the school health and nutrition initiative in Mangochi district, Malawi. Save the Children US , Malawi Country Office

[13] Mbah, M. & Useh, M. F. (2008). The relationship between urinary schistosomiasis and the prevailing socio-economic factors of a rural community in Cameroon. *Nigerian Journal of Parasitology*, 29.1, 5-1

[14] Ejezie, G. C. (1983). The Nigerian environment and parasitic infections. *Folia Parasitologica* (PRAHA), 30: 89-95

[15] Wernsdorfer, W. H. (1976). Malaria. World Health Organization working document. TDR/WP 76.6

[16] Edungbola, L. D., Asaolu, S. O., Omonisi, M. K. & Aiyedun, B. A. (1988). S. *haematobium* infection among children in Babana district, Kwara State. *African Journal of Medical Science*, 4.4,187-193.

[17] Useh, M. F. & Ejezie, G. C. (1996). Prevalence and morbidity of *S haematobium* infection in Adim community of Nigeria. *Journal of Medical Laboratory Science*, 5, 10-15

[18] Useh M. F. & Ejezie, G. C. (1999b). School-based schistosomiasis control programme: a comparative study on the prevalence and intensity of urinary schistosomiasis among Nigerian school-age children in and out of school. *Transactions of the Royal Society of Tropical Medicine and Hygiene*, 93, 387-391

[19] Akinwale, O. P., Ajayi, M.B., Akande, D. O., Gyang, P. V., Adeleke, M. A., Adeneye, A. K., Adebayo, M. O. & Dike, A. A. (2010). Urinary schistosomiasis around Oyan Reservoir, Nigeria: Twenty years after first outbreak. *Iranian J Public Health*, 39.1, 92-95.

[20] Banji, B. B., Mann, A., Nma, E., Obi, P. U. & Ezeako, I. A. (2011). Prevalence of schistosomiasis and other intestinal helminth parasites among school children in Bida, Niger State, Nigeria. *European Journal of Scientific Research*, 48.4, 621-626

[21] Goselle, N. O., Anegbe, D., Imandeh, G. N., Dakul, D. A., Onwuliri, A. C. F., Abba, O. J., Udeh, O. E. & Abelau, A. M. (2010). *Schistsoma haematobium* infections among school children in Jos, Nigeria. *Science World Journal*, 5.1,42-45

[22] Akufongwe, P. F., Dakul, D. A., Michael, P. D., Dajagat, P. D. & Arabs, W. L. (1996). Urinary schistosomiasis in rural communities of some local government areas in Plateau State, Nigeria: a preliminary parasitological and malacological survey. *Journal of Helminthology*, 70.1, 3-6.

[23] Ekpo, U. F., Akintunde, L., Akinola, S. O., Sam-Wobo, S. O. & Mafiana, C. F. (2010). Urinary schistosomiasis among preschool children in a rural community near Abeokuta, Nigeria. *Parasites and Vectors*,3:58

[24] Chugh, K. S., Harries, A. D., Dahniya, M. H., Nwosu, A. C., Gashau, A., Thomas, J. O., Thaliza, T. D., Hegger, S. & Onwuchekwa, A. C. (1986). Schistosomiasis in Maiduguri, north east, Nigeria. *Ann. Tropical Medicine and Parasitology*, 80.6, 593-99

[25] Pugh, R. N. H., Bell, D. R. & Gilles, H. M. (1980). Malumfashi endemic diseases research project, XV. The potential medical importance of bilharziasis in northern Nigeria. a suggested rapid, cheap and effective solution for control of *S haematobium* infection. *Annals of Tropical Medicine & Parasitology*, 74, 597-613

[26] Lichtenberg, Von F., Sher, A., Gibbons, N., Doughty, B. L. (1976). Eosinophil-enriched inflammatory response to schistosomula in the skin of mice immune to *S mansoni*. *American Journal of Pathology*, 84, 479-500

[27] Gilles, H. M., Lucas, A., Adeniyi, J. C., Lindner, R., Anand, S. V., Braband, H., Cockshott, W. P., Cowper, S. G., Muller, R. L., Hira, P. R. & Wilson, A. M. M. (1965). *Schistosoma haematobium* infection in Nigeria. 11. Infection at a primary school in Ibadan. *Annal of Tropical Medicine and Parasitology*, 59, 441-50

[28] Attah, Ed. 'B. (2000). Human Pathology- A complete text for Africa. Ibadan University Press, Ibadan, Nigeria, 198-202.

[29] Meremikwu, M. M., Asuquo, P.N., Ejezie, G. C., Useh, M. F. & Udoh, A. E. (2000). Treatment of *S haematobium* with praziquantel in children: its effect on educational performance in rural Nigeria. *Tropical Medicine*, 39-45.

[30] Ejezie, G. C. & Ade-Serrano, M. A. (1981b). *Schistosoma haematobium* in Ajara community of Badagry, Nigeria. Metrifonate trials in the treatment of the disease. *Tropical Geographical Medicine*, 33,181-184.

[31] Ekanem, E. E., Asindi, A. A., Ejezie, G. C. & Antia-Obong, O. E. (1994). Effect of *S. haematobium* infection on the physical growth and school performance of Nigerian children. *Central African Journal of Medicine*, 40.2, 30-44.

[32] Corbet, E. L., Butterworth, A. E., Fulford, A. J. C., Ouma, J. H.& Sturrock, R. F. (1992). Nutritional status of children with schistosomiasis mansoni in two different areas of Machakos district, Kenya. *Transactions of the Royal Society of Tropical Medicine and Hygiene*, 86, 266-273.

[33] Stephenson, L. S., Latham, M. C., Kurz, K. M., Kinotic, S. N., Oduori, M. L & Crompton, D. W (1985). Relationships of *S haematobium*, hookworm and malaria infections and metrifonate treatment to growth of Kenyan schoolchildren. *American Journal of Tropical Medicine and Hygiene*,34,1109-1118.

[34] Stephenson, L. S., Latham, M. C., Kurz, K. M., Kinotic, S. N.(1989). Single dose metrifonate or praziquantel treatment in Kenyan children. 11. effects on growth in relation

to S haematobium and hook egg counts. *American Journal of Tropical Medicine and Hygiene*,41, 445-453.

[35] Feldmeier, H., Poggensee, G & Krantz, I. (1993). A synoptic inventory of needs for research on women and tropical parasitic diseases. 11. Gender-related biases in the diagnosis and morbidity assessment of schistosomiasis in woman. *Acta Tropica*, 55, 139-169

[36] Weiland, G. (1989). The significance of immunodiagnosis in schistosomiasis control- a brief review. *Annal Tropical Medicine & Parasitology*

[37] World Health Organisation (1991). Ultrasound in the assessment of pathological changes. TDR/SCH/Ultrasound/913,2-6

[38] World Health Organisation (1978). Schistosomiasis. Technical Report Series, World Health Organisation, No 515, 1-47

[39] Mott, K. E. (1983). A reusable polyamide filter for diagnosis of *Schistosoma haematobium* infection by urine filtration. *Bull de la Soc. De Path Exotique*, 76, 101-104.

[40] Ejezie, G. C. & Ade-Serrano, M. A. (1981a). *Schistosoma haematobium* in Ajara community of Badagry. A study on prevalence, intensity and morbidity of infection among primary school children. *Tropical Geographical Medicine*, 37, 175-180.

[41] Smith, J. H., Kamel, I. A., Elwi, A., Lichtenberg, F. (1974). A quantitative post mortem analysis of urinary schistosomiasis in Egypt. 1. pathology and pathogenesis. *American Journal of Tropical Medicine & Hygiene*, 23, 1054-71

[42] Feldmeier, H., Doehring, E. & Daffalla, A. A. (1982). Simultaneous use of a sensitive filtration technique and reagent strips in urinary schistosomiasis. *Transactions of the Royal Society of Tropical Medicine & Hygiene*, 76.3, 416-421

[43] Ebrahim, A., El Morshedy, H., Omer, E., El Daly, S & Barakat, R (1997). Evaluation of the kato-katz smear and formol ether sedimentation techniques for the quantitative diagnosis of *S mansoni* infection. *American Jorunal of Tropical Medicine and Hygiene*, 57, 706-708

[44] Van Etten, L., Kremsner, P. G., Krijger, F. W. & Deelder, A. M. (1997). Day-to-day variation of egg output and schistosome circulating antigens in urine of *S haematobium*-infected school children from Gabon and follow up after chemotherapy. *Americal Journal of Tropical Medicine and Hygiene*, 57, 337-341.

[45] Ye, X. P., Donnelly, C. A., Anderson, R. M. Fu, Y. L., & Agnew, A. M. (1998). The distribution of *S japonicum* eggs in faeces and the effect of stirring faecal specimens. *Annals of Tropical Medicine and Parasitology*, 92, 181-185

[46] Cheever, A. W. (1968). A quantitative post-mortem study of schistosomiasis mansoni in man. *Americal Journal of Tropical Medicine and Hygiene*, 17, 38-64

[47] Agnew, A. M., Murare, H.M., Sandoval, S. N., De jong, N., Krijer, F. W., Deelder, A. M. & Doenhoff, M. J (1992). The susceptibility of adult schistosomes to immune attrition. *Memorias do Instituto Oswaldo Cruz,* 87 (S4), 87-93

[48] Leiter, J (1880). Beschreibung and Instruction Zur Handhabung der Von Dd. M. Nitze and Leite Construierten Instruments and Apparate wehelm Braumuller son, wein.

[49] Onyediran, A. B. O. O., Abayomi, I. O., Akinkugbe, O. O., Bohrer, S. P. & Lucas, A. (1975). Renographic studies in vesical schistosomiasis in children. *American Journal of Tropical Medicine & Hygiene,* 24, 274-279

[50] Hatz, C., Jenkins, J. M., Mendt, R., Wahab-Abdel, M. F. & Tanner, M. (1992). A review of the literature on the use of ultrasonography with special reference to its use in field studies. 1. *Schistosoms haematobium. Acta Tropica,* 51.1, 1-14.

[51] Woodruff, L. & Bell, A. (1978). *A synopsis of infection and tropical diseases.* Henry King LTD, Dorchester, 156-161

[52] Bilharz, T. (1852). Weitre Beobachtungen uber *Distomum haematobium* I der pfortader des Menschen and Zum Zusammenhang mit bestimmten pathologischen Veranderungen. *Zeitchrift fur wissenschadftliche Zoologie,* 4, 72-76

[53] Ezzat, E., Osman, R A., Ahmet, K. Y & Soothill, J. F. (1974). The association between *Schistosoma haematobium* infection and heavy proteinuria. *Transactions of the Royal Society of Tropical Medicine & Hygiene,* 68, 315-318

[54] Greenham, R. & Cameron, A. H. (1980). *Schistosoma haematobium* and the nephrotic syndrome. *Transactions of the Royal Society of Tropical Medicine & Hygiene,* 74, 609-613

[55] Wilkins, H. A., Goll, P., De C. Marshal & Moore, P (1979). The significance of proteinuria and haematuria in *S haematobium* infection. *Transactions of the Royal Society of Tropical Medicine and Hygiene.*73,74-80

[56] Chugh, K. S. & Harries, A. D. (1983). *S. haematobium* infection and proteinuria. *Lancet,* 2, 583-585

[57] Farid, Z., Minner, W. F., Higashi, G. I. & Hassan, A. (1976) Reversibility of lesions in schistosomiasis: a brief review. *Journal of Tropical Medicine & Hygiene,* 9, 164-166

[58] Doehring, E., Ehrich, J. H. H., Vester, U., Feldmeier, H. Poggensee, U. & Brodehl, J. (1985). Proteinuria, haematuria and leucocyturia in children with mixed urinary and intestinal schistosomiasis. *Kidney International,* 28, 520-25

[59] Mott, K. E., Dixon, H., Ossei-Tutu, E. & England, E. C. (1985). Evaluation of reagent strips in urine tests for detection of *S haematobium* infection. A comparative study in Ghana and Zambia. *Bulletin of the World Health Organization,* 63, 125-133.

[60] Tanner, M., Holzer, E., Marti, H. P., Saladin, B & Degremont, A. A. (1983). frequency of haematuria and proteinuria among *S haematobium* infected children of two communities from Liberia and Tanzania. *Acta Tropica,* 40, 231-37

[61] Inyang-Etoh, P. C., Ejezie, G. C., Useh, M. F. (2005). Assessment of haematuria and proteinuria as diagnostic markers for monitoring treatment of urinary schistosomiasis with artesunate. *Mary Slessor Journal of Medicine*, 5.1, 1-4.

[62] Feldmeier, H. & Krantz, I (1993). A synoptic inventory of needs for research on women and tropical parasitic diseases. 1. Application to urinary and intestinal schistosomiasis. *Acta Tropica*, 117-138.

[63] Friedberg, D., Berry, A. V. & Schneider, J. (1991). Schistosomiasis of the female genital tract. *SAMJ, Suppl*, 3, 1-15.

[64] Hatz, C., Savioli, L., Mayourbanam, C., Ohunputh, J., Kisumkpa, U. M. & Tanner, M. (1990). Measurement of schistosome-related morbidity at community level in areas of different endemicity. *Bulletin of the World Health Organization*, 68.6, 777-87.

[65] Vester, U., Hertsch, M. & Ehrich, J. H. H. (1991). Examination of urine samples for circumcised and non-circumcised Sudanese girls and women. *Tropical Medicine & Parasitology*, 42, 237-242

[66] Puschel, E. (1988). Die Menstruation and Ihre Tabus. Ethnologie and Kulturelle. Bedeutung, New York

[67] Chitsulo. L., Lengeler, C. & Jenkins, J. (1995). Guide for the rapid identification of communities with a high prevalence of urinary schistosomiasis. UNDP/World Bank/ WHO TDR/SER/MSR/95.2, 1-30.

[68] Kroeger, A (1983). Health interview surveys in developing countries. A review of the methods and results. *International Journal of Epidemiology*, 12.4, 465-81

[69] Ross, D. A. & Vaughan, P. (1986). Health interview surveys in developing countries: A methodical reviews. Studies in *Family Planning*, 17.2, 78-94

[70] Tanner, M. (1989). Evaluation and monitoring of schistosomiasis control. *Tropical Medicine & Parasitology*, 40, 207-13

[71] Lengeler, C., Sala-Diakanda, O. & Tanner, M. (1992). Using questionnaires and existing administrative system: a new approach to health interviews. *Health Policy & Planning*, 7, 10-21

[72] Useh, M. F. & Ejezie, G. C. (2004). Evaluation and validation of the Questionnaire approach for the diagnosis of urinary schistosomiasis among Nigerian school pupils. *Mary Slessor Journal of Medicine*, 4, 63-71

[73] Lengeler, C., de Savingny, D., Mshinda, H., Mayombana, C., Tayari, S., Hatz, C., Dregmont, A. & Tanner, M. (1991). Community-based questionnaires and heath statistics as Tools for the cost-effective identification of communities at risk of schistosomiasis. *International Journal of Epidemiology*, 20, 796-807

[74] Hamilton, J. V., Klinkert, M. & Doenhoff, M. J. (1998). Diagnosis of schistosomiasis: antibody detection, with notes on parasitological and antigen detection methods. *Parasitology*, 117, S41-57

[75] Doenhoff, M. J., Butterworth, A. E., Hayes, R. J., Sturrock, R. F., Ouma, J. H., Koech, D., Prentice, M. & Bain, J. (1993). Sero-epidemiology and serodiagnosis of schistosomiasis in Kenya using crude and purified egg antigen in ELISA. *Transaction of the Royal Society of Tropical Medicine* & *Hygiene*, 87, 42-48.

[76] Kamal, K. D., Shaheen, H. I. & El-Said, A. A. (1994). Applicability of ELISA on buffer-eluates of capillary blood spotted on filter papers for the diagnosis and clinical staging of human schistosomiasis. *Tropical Geographical Medicine*, 46.3, 138-141.

[77] MacLaren, M. L., Draper, C. C., Roberts, J. M., Mintergoedbloed, E., Ligthart, G. S., Teesdale, C. H., Amin, M. A., Omer, A. H. S., Bartlett, A. & Voller, A. (1978). Studies on ELISA test for *S mansoni* infections. *Annals of Tropical Medicine & Parasitology*, 72, 243-253.

[78] Chan, M. A., Chiodini, P. L. & Doenhoff, M. J. (2010). Development of a new assay for the diagnosis of schistosomiasis, using cercarial antigens. *Transactions of the Royal Society of Tropical Medicine & Hygiene*, 104,255-258.

[79] De Jonge, N., Kremsner, P. G., Krijger, F. W., Schommer, G., Fillie, Y. E., Kornelis, D., Van Zeyl, R. J. M., Van Dam, G. J., Feldmeier, H & Deelder, A. M. (1990). Detection of schistosome circulating cathodic antigen by ELIZA using biotinylated monoclonal antibodies. *Transaction of the Royal Society of Tropical Medicine* & *Hygiene*, 87, 42-48.

[80] Bosempem, K. M., Asigbee, J., Otchere, J., Hanina, A., Kpo, K. H. & Kojima, S (1998). Accuracy of diagnosis of urinary schistosomiasis: comparison of parasitological and a monoclonal antibody-based dipstick method. *Parasitology International*, 47, 211-217

[81] Gemmel, M. A., Lawson, B. D. & Roberts, M. G. (1986). Control of echinococcus/ hydatidosis: Present status of the world wide progress. *Bulletin of the World Health Organisation*, 64, 313-323

[82] Davis, A. (1981). Principles of schistosomiasis control in relation to community health care. *Arneim Forsch* 31(1), 616-618

[83] King, C. H. (2009). Towards the elimination of schistosomiasis. *New England Journal of Medicine*, 360(2), 106-109

[84] Kloos, H. (1985). Water resources development and schistosomiasis ecology in the Awash Valley, Ethiopia. *Social Science and Medicine*, 17(9), 545-562.

[85] Useh, M. F. (2011). Control of schistosomiasis. In *Schistosomiasis*, eds Mohammad Bagher Rokni, INTECH Publishers, Croatia, 73-102

[86] Sulaiman, S. M., Traore, M., Engels, D., Hagan, P & Cioli, D. (2001). Counterfeit Praziquantel. *Lancet*. 358, 666-667.

[87] Andrews, P. (1981). Preclinical data of praziquantel. A summary of the efficacy of praziquantel against schistosomes in animal experiments and notes on its mode of actions. *Arzneim Forsch Res* 31(1), 538-541

[88] Doenhoff, M. J., Cioli, D. & Utzinger, J. (2008). Praziquantel: mechanisms of action, resistance and new derivatives for schistosomiasis. *Current Opinions in Infectious Diseases*, 21: 659-667.

[89] Doenhoff, M. J., Hagan, P., Cioli, D., Southgate, V., Pica-Mattocca, L., Botros, S., Coles, G., Tchuem, L. A. Mbaye, A. and Engels, D. (2009). Praziquantel: its use in control of schistosomiasis in sub-saharan Africa and current research needs. *Parasitology*, 136, 1825-1835.

[90] Jeziorski, M. C. & Greenberg, R. M. (2006). Voltage-gated calcium channel subunits from platyheminths: potential role in praziquantel action. *American Journal of Tropical Medicine and Hygiene*, 36, 625-632.

[91] Pica-Mattoccia, L., Orsini, T., Basso, A., Festucci, A., Liberti, P., Guidi, A., Marcatto-Maggi, A. L., Nobre-Santana, S., Troiana, A. R., Cioli, D. & Valle, C. (2008). *Schistosoma mansoni*: lack of correlation between praziquantel-induced intra-worm calcium influx and parasite death. *Experimental Parasitology*, 119,332-335

[92] Pax, R., Bennett, J. L.& Fetterer, R. (1978). A benzodiazine derivative and praziquantel: effects on musculature of *S. mansoni* and *S. japonicum*. *Naunyn-Schiedbergs Arch Pharmacol*, 304, 309-315

[93] Doenhoff, M. J., Sabah, A. A., Fletcher, C., Webbe, G. & Bain, J. (1987). Evidence for an immune dependent action of praziquantel on *Schistosoma mansoni* in mice. *Transactions of the Royal Society Medicine and Hygiene*. 81, 947-951.

[94] Angelucci, F., Basso, A., Bellelli, A *et al* (2007). The antischistosomal drug praziquantel is an adenosine antagonist. *Parasitology*, 134: 1215-1221.

[95] Utzinger, J., Keiser, J., Xiao, S. H., Tanner, M. & Singer, B. H. (2003). Combination therapy of schistosomiasis in laboratory studies and clinical trials. *Antimicrobial Agents and Chemotherapy*, 47, 1487-1495.

[96] Secor, W. E. & Colley, D. G. (2005). Schistosomiasis. Springer Science and Business Media Incoporated, New York, USA.

[97] Danso-Appiah, A., Utzinger, J., Liu, J & Olliaro, P (2008). Drugs for treating urinary schistosomiasis. Cochrane Database System Review.

[98] Mgeni, A. F., Kisumku, U. M., McCullough, F. S., Dixon, H., Yoon, S. S. & Mott, K. E. (1990). Metrifonate in the control of urinary schistosomiasis in Zanzibar. *Bulletin of the World Health Organisation*, 68(6), 721-730

[99] Hommel, M. (2008). The future of artemisinins: natural, synthetic or recombinant. *Journal of Biology*, 7(10): Hommel, M. (2008). The future of artemisinins: natural, synthetic or recombinant. Journal of Biology, 7(10),38-42.

[100] Allen, H. E., Crompton, D. W. T., de Silva, N., LoVerde, P. T. & Olds, G. R. (2002). New policies for using anthelmintics in high risk Group. *Trends in Parasitology* , 18, 381-382

[101] Xiao, S. H., Keiser, J, Chollet, J *et al* (2007). In vitro and invivo activities of synthetic trioxolanes against major human schistosome species. *Antimicrobial Agents &Chemotherapy*, 51, 1440-1445

[102] Inyang-Etoh, P. C., Ejezie, G. C., Useh, M. F. & Inyang-Etoh, E (2009). Efficacy of a combination of praziquantel and artesunate in the treatment of urinary schistosomiasis in Nigeria. *Transactions of the Royal Society of Tropical Medicine and Hygiene*, 103, 38-44

[103] Inyang-Etoh, P. C., Ejezie, G. C., Useh, M. F. & Inyang-Etoh, E (2004). Efficacy of artesunate in the treatment of urinary schistosomiasis in an endemic community in Nigeria. *Annals of Tropical Medicine and Parasitology*, 98.5, 491-499.

[104] Richards, F. O., Eigege, A., Miri, E. S., Jinadu, M. Y. & Hopkins, D. R.(2006). Integration of mass drug administration programmes in Nigeria: the challenge of schistosomiasis. *Bulletin of World Health Organisation*, 84(8), 673-677

[105] Ottesen, E. A. (2002). Major progress towards eliminating lymphatic filariasis. *New England Journal of Medicine*, 247, 1885-6

[106] Savioli, L., Stansfield, S., Bundy, D. A., Mitchell, A., Bhatia, R., Engels D. et al (2002). Schistosomiasis and soil-transmitted helminth infections: forging control efforts. *Transactions of the Royal Society of Tropical Medicine and Hygiene*,96, 577-9

[107] Chitsulo, L., Engels, D., Montressor, A. & Savioli, L (2000). The global status of schistosomiasis and its control. *Acta Tropica*, 77(1), 41-51

[108] El Khoby, T., Galal, N., Fenwick, A. (1998). The UASID/government of Egypt's schistosomiasis research Project. *Parasitology Today*, 14, 92-96

[109] Hopkins, D. R., Eigege, S. & Miri, E. S. *et al* (2002). Lymphatic filariasis elimination and schistosomiasis control in combination with onchocerciasis control in Nigeria. *American Journal of Tropical Medicine & Hygiene*, 67, 266-272

[110] Na-Bangchang, K., Kietinun, S., Pawa, K. K., Hanpitakpong, W., Na-Bangchang, C & Lazdins, J. (2006). Assessment of pharmacokinetic drug interactions and tolerability of albendazole, praziquantel and ivermectin combination. *Transactions of the Royal Society of Tropical Medicine and Hygiene*, 100: 335-45

[111] Atun, R. *et al* (2010). Integration of targeted intervention into health systems: a conceptual framework for analysis. *Health Policy and Planning*, 25(2), 104-111.

[112] De Savigny, D & Adam T. (2009). Systems. Thinking for health systems strengthening, Geneva, WHO.

[113] Mahoney, R. T. & Morel, C. M. (2006). A global health innovations system. *Innovation Strategy Today*, 2(1), 1-12

[114] Coles, G. C., Bruce, J. I., Kinotic, G. K., Muttahi, W. T., Dias, J. C. S., Rocha, R. S. & Katz, N. (1987). The potential for drug resistance in schistosomiasis. *Parasitology Today*, 3, 34-38.

[115] Butterworth, A. E., Dunne, D. W., Fulford, A. J. C., Thorne, K.J. I., Gachuhi, K., Ouma, J. H & Sturrock, R. K (1992). Human immunity to *S. mansoni*: Observations on mechanisms and implications for control. *Immunological Investigations*, 21(5), 391-407.

[116] Lehman, J. S., Mott, K. E., Morrow, R. H., Muniz, T. M. & Boyer, M. H. (1976). The intensity and effects of infection with *S. mansoni* in a rural community in north East Brazil. *American Journal of Tropical Medicine and Hygiene*, 25, 285-294

[117] Chen, M. G. & Mott, K. E. (1989). Progress in assessment of morbidity due to schistosomiasis. *Tropical Disease Bulletin*, 86, 1-56

[118] Wilson, R. A. and Coulson, P. A. (2006). Schistosome vaccines: a critical appraisal. *Mem Inst Cruz Rio de Janeiro*, 10(Suppl.10), 13-20.

[119] Sadun, E. H. and Lin, S. S. (1959). Studies on the host parasite relationship to *S. japonicum*. IV. Resistance acquired by infection, by vaccination and by the injection of immune serum, in monkeys, rabbits and mice. *Journal of Parasitology*, 45, 543-54

[120] Murrell, K. D., Dean, D. A. & Stafford, E. E. (1975). Resistance to infection with *S. mansoni* after immunization with worm extracts or live cercarial: role of cyctotoxic antibody in mice and guinea pig. *American Journal of Tropical Medicine and Hygiene*, 24, 955-962

[121] Smithers, S. R. & Terry, R. J. (1969). Immunity in schistosomiasis. *Annals of NewYork Academy of Science*,160,826-840.

[122] Kariuki, T. M., Farah, I. O., Yole, D. S., Mwenda, J.M., Van Dam, G. J., Deelder, A. M., Wilson, R. A. & Coulson, P. S. (2004). parameters of attenuated schistosome vaccine evaluated in the olive baboon. *Infection and Immunology*. 72, 5526-5529.

[123] Coulson, P.S & Kariuki, T. M. (2006). Schistosome vaccine testing: lessons from the baboon model. *Mem Inst Oswaldo Cruz, Rio de janeiro*, 101(Suppl.1): 369-372.

[124] Capron, A., Capron, M & Riveau, G. (2002). Vaccine development against schistosomiasis from Concepts to clinical trials. *British Medical Bulletin*, 62, 139-148.

[125] Capron, A., Riveau, G., Capron, M. & Trottein, F (2005). Schistosomes: the road from host-parasite interactions to vaccines in clinical trials. *Trends in Parasitology*, 21:143-149.

[126] Curwen, R. S., Ashton, P. D., Johnston, D. A. & Wilson, R. A. (2004). The *S. mansoni* soluble protein: a comparison across four life-cycle stages. *Molecular Biochemistry and Parasitology*,138, 57-66.

[127] Dillon, G. P., Feltwell, T., Skelton, J. P., Ashton, P. D., Coulson, P. S., Quail, M. A., Nikolaidou-Katsaridou, N, Wilson, R. A. & Ivens, A. C. (2006). Microarray analysis identifies genes preferentially expressed in the lung schistosomulum of *S. mansoni*. *International Journal of Parasitology*,36, 1-8

Section 2

Clinical Schistosomiasis

Chapter 5

Clinical, Laboratory and Ultrasonographic Evaluation of Patients with Acute Schistosomiasis Mansoni

Matheus Fernandes Costa-Silva**,
Denise da Silveira-Lemos**,
Amanda Cardoso de Oliveira Silveira,
Pedro Henrique Gazzinelli-Guimarães,
Helena Barbosa Ferraz, Cristiano Lara Massara,
Martin Johannes Enk,
Maria Carolina Barbosa Álvares,
Olindo Assis Martins-Filho,
Paulo Marcos Zech Coelho, Rodrigo Corrêa-Oliveira,
Giovanni Gazzinelli and Andréa Teixeira-Carvalho

Additional information is available at the end of the chapter

http://dx.doi.org/10.5772/53047

1. Introduction

Schistosomiasis is a parasite chronic disease caused by the helminth of genus *Schistosoma*. The infection is common in parts of Africa, South America, Middle East, Caribbean and Asia where it is a leading cause of morbidity and mortality [1]. Recent estimates suggest there are 700 million people at risk worldwide with almost 200 million infected in Africa alone [2]. In Brazil, the schistosomiasis infection is caused by *Schistosoma mansoni,* where estimates suggest a range from 2.5 million [3, 4] to 12 million people infected [5]. In the state of Minas Gerais, schistosomiasis mansoni is prevalent in 519 out of 853 municipalities, with an estimated number of one million infected people in an area of 300.000 km^2 [6].

One of the greatest public health problems in countries where the disease is highly endemic, including Brazil, is schistosomiasis control for the following reasons: (a) large intermediary hosts dissemination and their escape mechanisms from molluscicides and from biological control due to high costs and low efficacy; (b) high charges associated with implementation of sanitary conditions and water supply and the intense contact of rural population with polluted water, as well as engagement in agricultural and fishing activities; (c) the long time needed for sanitary education and for the community to adhere to controlling programs; (d) individual or massive treatment has been shown efficient for controlling the morbidity, but not for reducing prevalence due to reinfection; (e) individual protection is unlikely, except for specific groups of exposed people; (f) until the current days, there is no effective vaccine for preventing schistosomiasis [7, 8].

According to previous data published by our group [9, 10], the proliferation of rural tourism in endemic areas may be an important contributing factor to the outbreak of schistosomiasis cases. The preservation of natural environment on the site, in order to attract visitors from urban centers, unintentionally contributes to create an ideal habitat for the intermediate host. Additionally, most areas chosen for leisure activities accommodate rural communities without any type of sanitation and, thus, represent a permanent risk of contamination of the flowing water.

In this context, visitors from urban areas, who never had previous contact with the parasite, contract the infection, and develop acute schistosomiasis [11]. Acute schistosomiasis is associated with a primary exposure and is more commonly seen in non-immune individuals traveling through endemic regions [12]. The clinical symptoms most commonly observed in such patients include fever, general weakness, headache, nausea, vomiting, diarrhea, anorexia, colic, weight loss, dry cough and hepatosplenomegaly accompanied by marked eosinophilia and leucocytosis [13-16]. However, these clinical symptoms may be confused with a number of infections such as visceral leishmaniasis, typhoid fever, malaria, tuberculosis, viral hepatitis, mononucleosis and bacterial infections [17]. Hence, the diagnosis of acute schistosomiasis becomes a challenge for the assistant doctor due to the wide diversity of non-specific symptoms presented by the patients; in addition, the presence of eggs in stool may not to be easily detected by parasitological examination in this phase of the infection.

Abdominal ultrasound is a complementary tool often used to assist the diagnoses of the *S. mansoni* infection, mainly on the study of the liver damage caused by the chronic infection. It is an inexpensive method, not radioactive or invasive, which provides immediate results and can be used for epidemiological fieldwork in endemic areas. The hepatic ultrasound pattern in patients with severe hepatosplenic schistosomiasis is characterized by pronounced periportal thickening. However, reports of ultrasound studies in patients with acute schistosomiasis are still scarce [18], and additional trials are necessary to evaluate the benefits and limitations of the ultrasound as a tool of clinical evaluation at the acute phase of the *S. mansoni* infection [19].

From the immunological point of view, the acute phase of the infection is characterized by a series of humoral and cellular immunological events. Hiatt et al. [20] showed elevations of IgG, IgM, IgE, and high titers of total antibodies in serum of acute patients that indicated the illness is associated with intense immune activity, while the magnitude of the IgE responses was related to the intensity of the infection. De Jesus et al. [16] showed that there was no significant difference in total IgE level between patients with acute and chronic schistosomiasis. In addition, Caldas et al [21] showed that specific IgG, IgM and IgE titers against egg and worm antigens in acute patients do not differ from those presented by chronic patients. Regarding cellular immunological events, nitric oxide (NO) represents an important and versatile messenger in biological systems, and it has been identified as a cytotoxic factor in the immune system, presenting anti- or pro-inflammatory properties under different circumstances [22]. Oliveira et al. [23] demonstrated that human peripheral blood mononuclear cells (PBMC) are capable of *in vitro* NO production and the inhibition of its production through the addition of N omega-nitro-L-arginine methyl ester (L-NAME) is responsible for an exacerbated granulomatous reaction.

In this report, we evaluated the clinical/laboratorial parameters and ultrasonographic features of patients who suffered acute schistosomiasis resulting from a simultaneous exposure in a country house in the metropolitan area of Belo Horizonte, Minas Gerais State, Brazil.

2. Population, materials and methods

2.1. Study population

The patients evaluated in this study acquired the acute phase of *S. mansoni* infection in a country house in the rural district of the municipality of Igarapé in the metropolitan area of Belo Horizonte, Brazil. The country house is frequently leased during the weekends and long holidays. It is a large house with a pool of water supplied by a stream. Beside the pool, the water from the stream was channeled into open channels to form a shower. During the inspection of the country house, researchers at the Research Center Rene Rachou (CPqRR) – Oswaldo Cruz Foundation, at the Brazilian Ministry of Health detected that the place did not have basic sanitation. All the water used was damped, discarded in a dam located near the house. Out of forty-two individuals who were in the country house, thirty-eight participated in the study and were previously evaluated. After a preliminary assessment, we found that nineteen infected patients had been treated previous to our evaluation and five patients did not fulfill the inclusion criteria described below. Therefore, these patients were excluded from the study apart from other four subjects who had negative stool examination for *S. mansoni*. Thus, the group of patients evaluated was composed by ten individuals, five women and five men, aging 14 to 31 years, with parasite load ranging from 8 to 768 eggs per gram of feces (epg).

To participate in the study, patients in the acute phase of schistosomiasis have fulfilled the following criteria for inclusion: age between 10 and 65 years; did not report having received any treatment with anti-helminthic drugs in the last 24 months; diagnosis of acute schistosomiasis mansoni based on epidemiological data (recent contact with *S. mansoni* cercariae-contaminated water), clinical symptoms (acute enterocolitis, nausea, vomiting, abdominal pain, fever, headache, weight loss, cough, cercarial dermatitis, hepatomegaly and splenomegaly) and laboratory data (eosinophilia and viable *S. mansoni* eggs in stool). Each volunteer or their legal guardian signed their informed consent. In addition, we also excluded from this study all patients who had one of the following conditions: unable to hold examinations proposed; alcoholism, defined as above average weekly consumption of 420 grams of ethanol (daily average over 60 g of ethanol) [24]; pregnancy, defined by laboratory criteria; significant anemia defined as hemoglobin less than 10 g/dl [25] and any other significant systemic disease, acute or chronic, that could interfere with the results of the proposed methods.

After blood collection, all patients who had positive stool examination for *S. mansoni*, regardless of participation in the study, were submitted to treatment with the standard Brazilian dose of Praziquantel (50-60 mg/kg).

A group of healthy volunteers formed by nine individuals, one woman and eight men aged 25 to 42 years, blood donors of the blood bank of Hospital Felicio Rocho, Belo Horizonte, Minas Gerais, Brazil constituted a control group (CT). It is important to mention that these individuals were screened and selected after serological tests for negativity for Chagas disease, leishmaniasis, human immunodeficiency virus (HIV), hepatitis, and did not report previous infection with *S. mansoni*.

The study was carried out according to the National Health Council resolution 196/96, which regulates the research involving human beings, and was approved by the Ethics Committees of the Faculty of Medicine, Federal University of Minas Gerais, Oswaldo Cruz Foundation, and the Brazilian National Committee on Ethics in Research.

2.2. Parasitological examination

Parasitological examination was performed using the Kato-Katz method [26]. The presence and the number of *S. mansoni* eggs per gram of feces were determined through examination of six blades per one stool sample for each patient. The results are presented as the arithmetic mean of number of eggs. The Kato-Katz method is the method of choice to measure infection level and has been used extensively in epidemiological studies.

2.3. Evaluation of clinical parameters

All the individuals who came into contact with water contaminated by cercariae were subjected to a detailed history, performed by a physician of our team. The survey used during this study contained data referring to number of the protocol, name, gender, age, education and place of birth and questions about the clinical symptoms/signs such as fever, diarrhea, nausea, vomiting, abdominal pain, cough, weight loss, headache, asthenia, facial edema and cercarial dermatitis.

2.4. Evaluation of hematological parameters

Peripheral blood was collected in 5 mL vacuum tubes containing ethylenediamine tetraacetic acid (EDTA) as anticoagulant (Vacutainer, Beckton Dickinson, CA, USA), approximately 40 days after contact with contaminated water by cercariae and only once prior to treatment with praziquantel. The hemograms were performed in automated hematological electronic counter (Coulter MD18, E.U.A). The parameters measured were hemoglobin, number of erythrocytes and hematocrit values as well as total and differential counts of leukocytes including absolute counts of eosinophils, neutrophils, lymphocytes and monocytes.

2.5. Total IgE measurement

The plasma levels of total IgE antibodies were quantified using *Colorimetric Immunoenzymatic kit* (SYM Total IgE, Symbiosis Diagnostic, Brazil). Aliquots of 25 μL of plasma and six standards (Reagent kit SYM Total IgE Symbiosis Diagnostic, Brazil) at concentrations of 0, 5, 25, 50, 150 and 400UI/mL were dispensed in duplicates in wells of flat-bottomed plates, previously sensitized with streptavidin, together with 100 μL of monoclonal anti-human IgE conjugated to biotin (Reagent kit SYM Total IgE Symbiosis Diagnostic, Brazil). The plates were incubated for 30 minutes at room temperature in the dark and washed five times with 300 μL/well of wash solution (Reagent kit SYM Total IgE Symbiosis Diagnostic, Brazil). Subsequently were added 100 μL of a second monoclonal anti-human IgE conjugated to peroxidase. The plates were incubated for 30 minutes at room temperature, in the dark, and washed five times with 300 μL/well of wash solution. Then, 100 μL of chromogen-substrate solution (tetramethylbenzidine-TMB) (Reagent kit SYM Total IgE Symbiosis Diagnostic, Brazil) were added by well, and the plate was incubated for 15 minutes in the dark. The reaction was stopped by adding 100 μL of 1N sulfuric acid (H2SO4) per well (Reagent kit SYM Total IgE Symbiosis Diagnostic, Brazil). The optical density of samples and standards was measured in an automatic reader (Molecular Devices Versa Max, California, USA) using a 450 nm filter.

2.6. Nitric oxide plasma levels

The plasma levels of nitric oxide were quantified using *Immunoenzymatic kit QuantiChromTM Nitric Oxide* (Quantitative Colorimetric Determination of Nitric Oxide, BioAssay Systems, USA). The assays were performed according to the manufacturer's recommendations. The deproteination of samples was made by adding 80 mL of zinc sulfate (ZnSO4) 75 mM final concentration and 120 mL of sodium hydroxide (NaOH) 55 mM final concentration. Samples were centrifuged at 400 g for 5 minutes at 4°C. Then 70 mL of glycine buffer was added in each sample. Afterwards, aliquots of 100 μL of plasma and eight standards at concentrations of 0, 5, 10, 15, 20, 30, 40 and 50 μM mL were dispensed in duplicates in 1.5 mL tubes. Then, samples were placed in the presence of cadmium activated with 200 mL of Buffer Activation and incubated for 15 minutes. The samples were transferred in duplicates to their respective wells in flat-bottomed plates and added to 50 mL of reagents A and B. The optical density of samples and standards was measured in an automatic reader (Molecular Devices Reader-Precision, USA) using a 540 nm filter.

2.7. Evaluation of hepatic enzymes

For the analysis of hepatic functions for the study group, plasma concentration of the enzymes ALT (alaline amino transferase), AST (aspartate amino transferase) and γ-GT (gamma-glutamyl transferase) were quantified by kinetic method using *ALT/GPT Liquiform, AST/GOT Liquiform and GAMA GT Liquiform kits* (Labtest Diagnostic, Brazil) in the device Wiener Lab Metrolab 2300 plus (Model CM-200). The results were expressed in UI/mL.

2.8. Ultrasonographic analysis

Ultrasonographic evaluation was performed using a Nemio SSA/550ª machine (Toshiba, Town, Japan) with a 3-MHz sector probe for patients ≥ 10 years old and a 5-MHz probe for patients under 10 years old. The group of healthy individuals non-infected with *S. mansoni* (CT group) consisted of twelve volunteers, paired by sex and age with the infected patients. Seven acute patients, three women and four men aged 14 to 31 years old have had ultrasonographic evaluation. All study population was examined by the same physician (MCBA). Liver size, portal-vein diameter, thickness of the central walls and peripheral portal branches, spleen size and splenic vein diameters were assessed as described [27, 28]. The liver was also examined for surface smoothness. Portal vein diameter was measured at its entrance into the liver and its bifurcation inside the liver. The spleen was evaluated by using oblique and longitudinal scanning of the left upper quadrant. The gallbladder was examined for wall thickness and stones. The periportal thickness was evaluated according to previous established criteria by [27-29].

2.9. Statistical analysis

The statistical analysis of the data was made through GraphPad PRISM® 5.00 software release for Windows (La Jolla, CA, USA). Student's t test was used for parametric data comparison between two groups, while for non-parametric data we used the Mann-Whitney test. In all cases, the data were considered significant at $P < 0.05$.

3. Results

3.1. Demographic data and intensity of S. mansoni infection

Out of forty-two people who were present in the country house, thirty-eight (90.5%) participated in this study and reported contact with water contaminated with cercariae. Out of these, thirty-four (89.5%) had eggs of *S. mansoni* in their feces and four (10.5%) were repeatedly negative. According to criteria previously mentioned, twenty-four patients were excluded from the study and ten patients were considered to be on an ongoing acute phase of schistosomiasis. In the acute group (ACT), there were no significant differences in age between females and males (23.0 ± 7.8 and 19.8 ± 4.5 years old, respectively, p value = 0.45) and the intensity of infection did not differ regarding gender, (205.6 ± 318.5 and 98.4 ± 70.7 eggs/g of feces, respectively, P value = 0.50). The ACT group presented parasite load ranging from 8 to 768 eggs per gram of feces (152.0 ± 224.7).

Parameter	Subjects		
	Total individuals	Evaluated individuals	Acute patients
Number of subjects (%)	42 (100%)	38 (90.5%)	10 (23.8%)
Age			
Range	01 - 65	01 - 65	14 - 31
Mean ± SD	22.4 ± 15.2	22.5 ± 15.5	21.4 ± 6.2
Median	21.5	20.5	22.5
Gender			
Female	25 (59.5%)	22 (57.9%)	05 (50.0%)
Male	17 (40.5%)	16 (42.1%)	05 (50.0%)
Parasitological Examination			
Negative	----	04 (10.5%)	0
Positive	----	34 (89.5%)	10 (100%)
Egg counts (eggs/g of feces)			
Range	----	0 - 768	8 - 768
Mean ± SD	----	50.8 ± 132.2	152.0 ± 224.7
Median	----	10.0	86.0

Table 1. Characterization of the study population

3.2. Clinical manifestations

The magnitude of clinical manifestations of schistosomiasis varies from light to severe intensity. Two patients showed serious clinical symptoms and required hospitalization due to the severity of the disease. The patients reported the onset of symptoms 20-30 days after water exposure. Headache and fever (60.0% and 50.0%, respectively) were the most common symptoms among patients, followed by diarrhea and weight loss (both 40.0%). Other clinical symptoms/signals were also recorded such as nausea/vomiting, abdominal pain, cough, asthenia, facial edema (each one with frequency of 30.0%) as well as urticaria and cercarial dermatitis (both 10.0%).

Table 2 highlights the main features observed in different human studies evaluating acute phase of schistosomiasis mansoni performed in distinct brazilian states such as Pernambuco,

Sergipe and Minas Gerais. Although in these studies the frequency of exposed/infected individuals was similar ranging 90-100% and the incubation period has also occurred in comparable times such 20-30 days, we have observed strongly heterogeneous symptoms between them. Nonetheless, our study demonstrated some similar clinical symptoms in comparison to those found by Barbosa et al. 2001b [30] like the frequency of fever (50.0% and 54.0%, respectively), cough (30.0% and 33.0%, respectively) and urticaria (10.0% and 8.0%, respectively). However, other parameters presented distinct results like the frequency of headache (60.0% and 33.0%, respectively) and diarrhea (40.0% and 25.0%, respectively).

Parameters	Barbosa Et Al. 2001a [15]	Barbosa Et Al. 2001b [30]	De Jesus Et Al. 2002 [16]	This Study
Number of patients	**11**	**12**	**31**	**10**
Site/State	Ilha de Itamaracá Pernambuco	Escada Pernambuco	Aracaju Sergipe	Igarapé Minas Gerais
Exposed/infected	92%	100%	92%	90%
Incubation period (days)	15-30	20	20-30	20-30
Headache	36%	33%	87%	60%
Fever	100%	54%	90%	50%
Diarrhea	64%	25%	81%	40%
Cough	91%	33%	91%	30%
Abdominal pain	64%	N.E.	93%	30%
Urticaria	18%	08%	N.E.	10%
Cercarial dermatitis	100%	N.E.	N.E.	10%
Hepatomegaly	75%	N.E.	35%	86%
Transaminases (increase)	36%	N.E.	38%	N.L.

N.E. - not evaluated

N.L. - normal levels

Table 2. Main features observed in different human studies evaluating the acute phase of schistosomiasis mansoni

3.3. Plasma levels of total IgE and nitric oxide

The plasma levels of total IgE and nitric oxide from the ACT group are illustrated in Figure 1. The analysis of the results showed that the ACT group presented a significant ($P < 0.05$) increase of these parameters as compared with the CT group.

3.4. Hematological profile

The main findings related to the hematological profile from the ACT group are illustrated in Figures 2 and 3. The analysis showed a significant reduction in the concentration of hemoglobin in the ACT group as well as an increase in the total leukocytes count as compared with the CT group. Increased total leukocytes were reflected in the absolute values of lymphocytes and eosinophils also increased in the ACT group as compared with the CT group. No significant difference was found between these two groups regarding other analyzed parameters such as number of erythrocytes, percentage of hematocrit, and absolute values of neutrophils and monocytes.

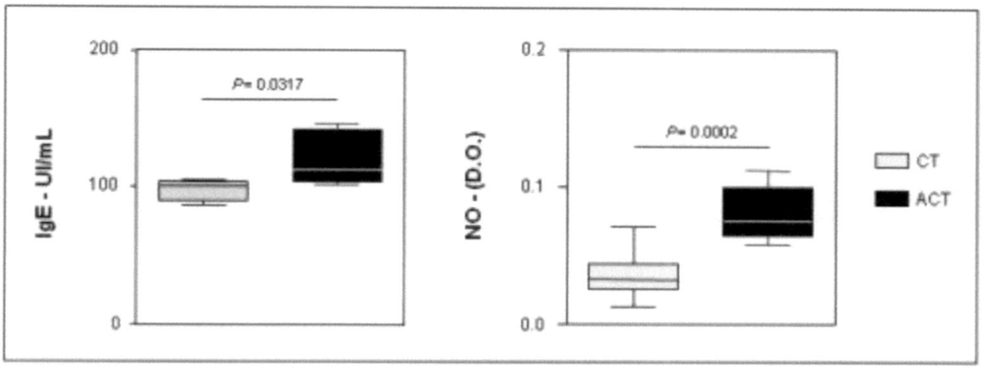

Figure 1. Total plasma IgE and nitric oxide (NO) levels in acute schistosomiasis patients (ACT=10) and non-infected individuals (CT=09). The results are expressed in box-plot format. The box stretches from the lower hinge (defined as the 25th percentile) to the upper hinge (the 75th percentile) and therefore contains the middle half of the scores in the distribution. The median is shown as a line across the box. Therefore 1/4 of the distribution is between this line and the top of the box and 1/4 of the distribution is between this line and the bottom of the box. Significant differences (connecting lines) were considered at $P < 0.05$.

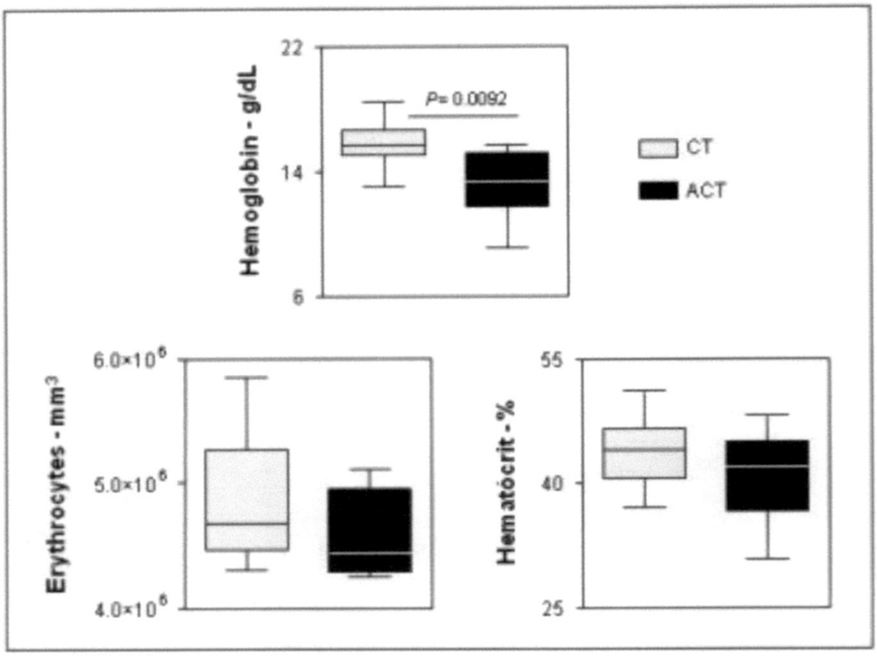

Figure 2. Hematological profile (hemoglobin-g/dL, erythrocytes/mm^3 and percentage of hematocrit) from acute schistosomiasis patients (ACT=10) and non-infected individuals (CT=09). The results are expressed in box-plot format. The box stretches from the lower hinge (defined as the 25th percentile) to the upper hinge (the 75th percentile) and therefore contains the middle half of the scores in the distribution. The median is shown as a line across the box. Therefore 1/4 of the distribution is between this line and the top of the box and 1/4 of the distribution is between this line and the bottom of the box. Significant differences (connecting lines) were considered at $P < 0.05$.

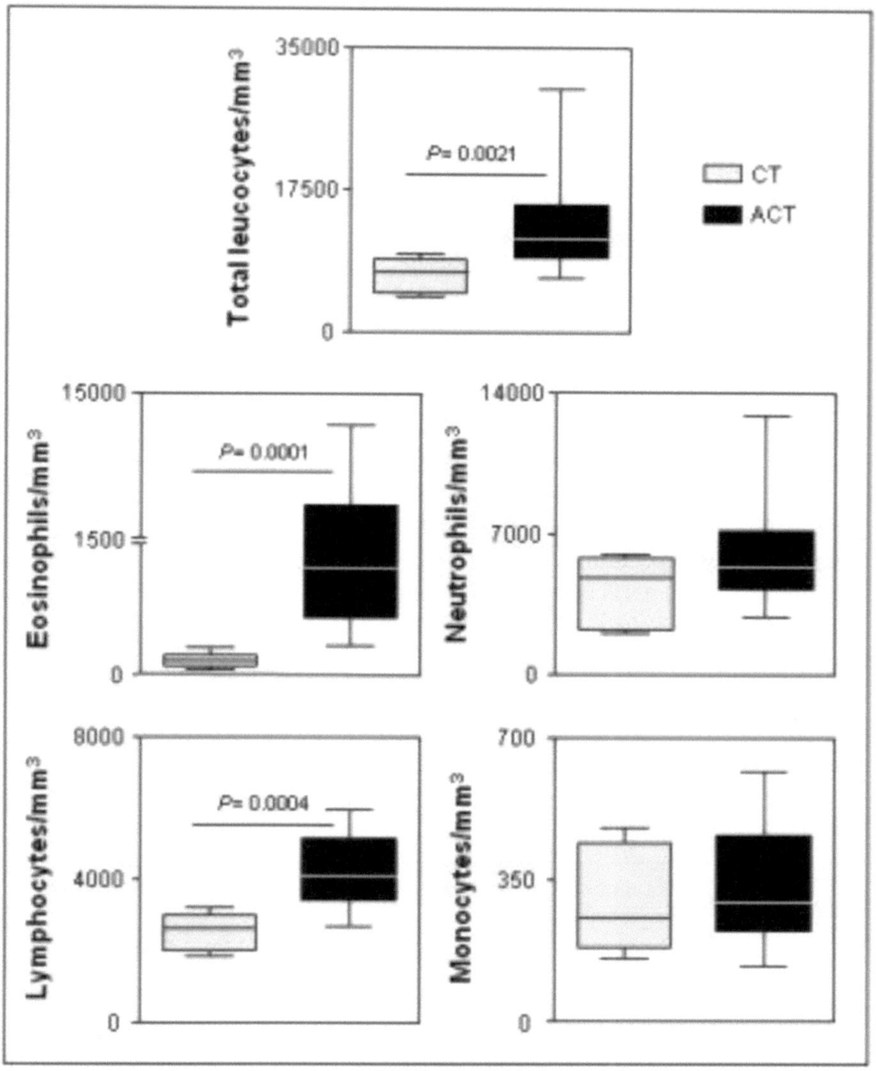

Figure 3. Total and differential leukocyte counts from acute schistosomiasis patients (ACT=10) and non-infected individuals (CT=09). The results are expressed in box-plot format highlighting the gap of 50% of data set measurement for absolute values in mm^3 of each leukocyte subset analyzed. Significant differences (connecting lines) were considered at $P < 0.05$.

3.5. Profile of hepatic enzymes

Acute patients presented levels of ALT, AST and γ-GT enzymes similar to reference values and there were no significant differences between these levels and those presented by CT group. (Table 3).

Hepatic Enzymes	Control Group (N = 9)	Acute Patients (N = 8)
ALT (alaline amino transferase) (3-50 U/mL)*	12.5 ± 11.2	8.6 ± 5.5
AST (aspartate amino transferase) (12-46 U/mL)*	18.7 ± 5.9	23.0 ± 6.7
γ-GT (gamma-glutamyl transferase) (9-61 U/L)*	23.4 ± 9.9	33.9 ± 16.6

Values are represented as mean ± standard deviation

* Reference values

Table 3. Hepatic serological tests in the study group

3.6. Ultrasonographic analysis

The results demonstrated that the ACT group presented some significant differences as compared with the CT group: medium increase in the measurement (in mm) of longitudinal left/right lobe of liver (117.4 ± 19.7 and 99.0 ± 12.3 or 150.1 ± 18.2 and 102.2 ± 16.0, respectively), size of longitudinal spleen (110.6 ± 16.3 and 91.2 ± 12.7, respectively) as well as dimension of Hilar portal vein wall (3.4 ± 1.0 and 1.5 ± 0.3, respectively) (Table 4). Periportal lymph node enlargement was observed in six of seven patients (85.7%). The periportal lymph nodes were larger, round or ovoid in shape and sharply defined with thin halos surrounding hypoechoic areas (Figure 4). An additional ultrasonographic feature observed was an incipient periportal echogenic thickening named as grade I fibrosis (Figure 5).

Site Of Measurement	Control Group (N = 12)	Acute Patients (N = 7)
Longitudinal left lobe of liver	99.0 ± 12.3	117.4 ± 19.7*
Anteroposterior left lobe of liver	46.7 ± 10.0	53.3 ± 10.9
Longitudinal right lobe of liver	102.2 ± 16.0	150.1 ± 18.2*
Anteroposterior right lobe of liver	68.6 ± 11.9	63.4 ± 9.6
Longitudinal spleen	91.2 ± 12.7	110.6 ± 16.3*
Anteroposterior spleen	35.1 ± 6.3	43.5 ± 11.1
Portal vein	10.0 ± 1.2	9.9 ± 1.9
Hilar portal vein wall	1.5 ± 0.3	3.4 ± 1.0*
Splenic vein	6.4 ± 1.3	7.1 ± 1.4
Superior mesenteric vein	6.7 ± 1.1	7.1 ± 1.3
Periportal lymph node	N.V.	1.8 ± 1.0*

Values are represented in mm as mean ± standard deviation

* Statistical difference ($p < 0.05$)

N.V. - not visualized (normal abdominal lymph nodes are usually not visualized by sonography)

Table 4. Ultrasonographic features of the study group

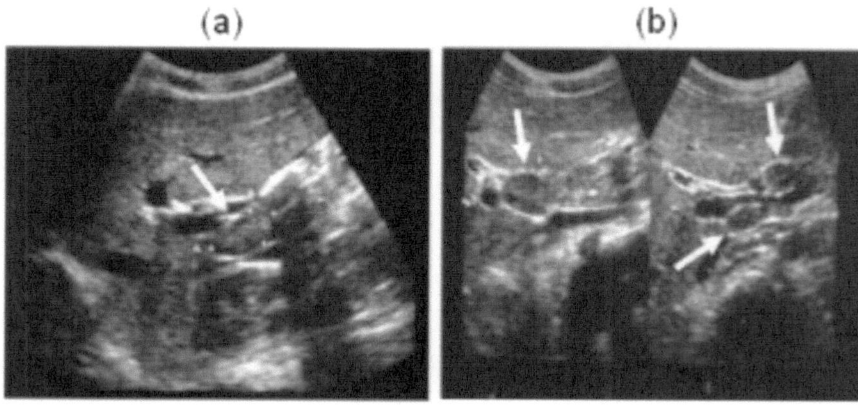

Figure 4. Representative ultrasonographic images of periportal lymph nodes from acute schistosomiasis patients. The arrows indicate larger lymph nodes, ovoid in shape (a) and rounded (b) with thin halos surrounding hypoechoic areas. Ultrasonographic analysis was performed with a Nemio SSA/550[a] machine (Toshiba).

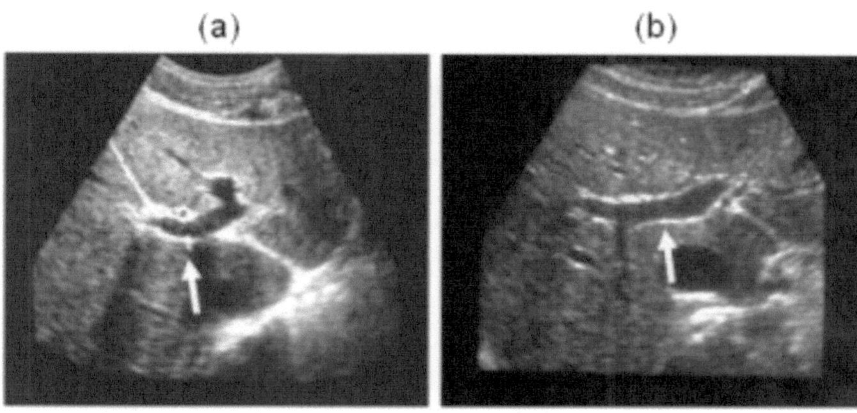

Figure 5. Representative ultrasonographic images of liver from acute schistosomiasis patient (a) and healthy volunteer (b). The arrows indicate incipient periportal echogenic thickening (a) and no periportal echogenic thickening (b). Ultrasonographic analysis was performed with a Nemio SSA/550[a] machine (Toshiba).

4. Discussion

The transmission of *S. mansoni* may vary depending on the ecology of the disease and the social standing of the population in which it occurs. The prevalence and intensity of the infection is subject to cultural practices, specific for each locality or situation and usually associated to economic, domestic or leisure activities [15, 31].

During the last decades, the traditional epidemiological pattern showed a tendency to change. Accelerating migration from the countryside to cities threatened to overwhelm existing water and sanitation systems, and to increase urban schistosomiasis [9, 32, 33]. In Brazil, especially in urban areas, acute schistosomiasis outbreaks were observed and documented with a certain frequency [9, 14, 15, 17, 34-36]. The increase of acute schistosomiasis cases also indicates that a non-immune fraction of the population became exposed to the disease [9, 10, 36].

The incidence of the acute form of schistosomiasis mansoni is certainly underestimated. This illness has been mainly described as a disease of travelers. Many scientific publications concerning this acute disease refer to groups of tourists, fishermen or sailors originally from a non-endemic country who have visited a tropical zone [17, 37, 38]. However, as schistosomiasis is a focally distributed infection [17, 39, 40], the acute form is also diagnosed in inhabitants from endemic countries who do not live in endemic areas. Nevertheless, acute disease is seldom recognized in infected patients from endemic areas. According to Lambertucci [41], acute schistosomiasis is most evident in primary infection in non-immune individuals. Among people living in endemic areas, the acute phase may pass undiagnosed. Because in endemic areas exposure to infection occurs early in life, symptoms would be inconspicuous and diagnosis not even suspected.

The clinical features of the acute phase of schistosomiasis mansoni present a wide spectrum [42, 43] and the relative contribution of host and parasite factors in the pathogenesis of the disease is not completely elucidated [20, 43-45]. According to Neves [46], the clinical forms of the disease will depend on the interaction of at least three sequential events: (a) the evolution phase of the worms, whether before or after oviposition and the deposition of eggs in the tissues; (b) the organ predominantly involved by young or mature worms and by their eggs; and (c) the type and the qualitative/quantitative deviation of the total and local host response to antigenic products derived from the disintegration of schistosomula, adult worms and their eggs.

The main clinical findings presented in our study such as headache, fever, diarrhea and weight loss were consistent with those found by other authors [9, 15-17]. Different intensities of clinical manifestation are observed in patients with acute schistosomiasis, some of them evolved with a relatively severe picture while others with mild symptoms. In our study, we have also observed a similar profile.

The development of non-apparent clinical form characterized by blood eosinophilia and a positive immediate cutaneous reaction in the initial phase of the *S. mansoni* infection was described by Rocha et al. [47]. According to previous data in the literature [13, 15, 16, 43], patients with acute phase of schistosomiasis in our study had an increased absolute number of eosinophils in comparison to reference data ranging between 400 to 600 cells/mm^3 [48]. Eosinophils are thought to play a major role in a variety of human diseases, including allergic inflammation, malignancy, and host defense against helminth infections. However, the exact role(s) of eosinophils in schistosomiasis regarding immunopathology remains unclear. Eosinophils may participate in Ab-dependent protective immune responses [49]. Human eosinophils express IgE receptors that participate in an IL-5-dependent Ab-dependent cell-mediated cytotoxicity reaction against schistosomula in vitro. Eosinophils also mediate the destruction of miracidia and schistosome eggs

[50]. Experimental studies have shown that the eosinophilia would be induced by type 2-cytokines as interleukin (IL)-4, IL-9, IL-13 and mainly by IL-5 [51]. According to Rocha et al. [43], the eosinophilia may be considered a possible pathogenic factor in acute schistosomiasis. The specific granules of the eosinophil contain lysosomal hydrolases as well as several cationic proteins like the major basic protein (MBP) [43, 52], the eosinophil cationic protein (ECP) and a neurotoxin, the eosinophil-derived neurotoxin (EDN), besides a peroxidase [43, 53]. The MBP in low concentrations is toxic to schistosomula but this action is non-selective since mammalian cells can also be damaged [43, 54, 55]. Both peroxidase and ECP are also toxic for helminths and mammal cells [43, 56, 57]. The cytolysis or eosinophil degranulation with the release of granule proteins can contribute to the genesis of local pathological alterations causing dysfunction or damage to the cells, especially when a great number of eosinophils are involved [43, 53, 58].

According to this report, acute patients presented increased plasma levels of IgE and nitric oxide as compared with the CT group. Our result is similar to the data published by De Souza et al. [59], which evaluated the humoral immune response through quantifying of the total IgE levels from patients with acute clinical form of schistosomiasis. Thus, we suggest that total IgE may be related to disease morbidity, as established by Pereira et al. [60]. Nitric oxide (NO) has been identified as an important cytotoxic factor and versatile messenger in the immune system being responsible to induce both anti- and/or proinflammatory effects [61]. There are broad direct and indirect evidences that NO can act as an anti-schistosomal and antiparasitic molecule [62-64]. Moreover, NO produced by human leukocytes has been shown to kill larval schistosome parasites [64, 65]. Studies in experimental models of acute schistosomiasis showed that the inhibition of iNOS resulted in cachexia and exacerbated hepatic pathology, suggesting that in schistosomiasis, NO limits hepatocyte damage [66-68].

From two to eight weeks after a first contact with natural water infested by *Schistosoma* cercariae, susceptible infected patients may present a syndrome comprising a period of 2 to 30 days of fever, diarrhea, toxemia and weakness, weight loss, abdominal pain, cough, mialgya, and arthralgia, edema, urticaria, nausea/vomiting and hepatosplenomegaly [7]. Until recently, acute schistosomiasis diagnosis was only based on epidemiological and clinical features, presence of *S. mansoni* eggs in stools and eosinophilia. However, the diagnosis becomes a challenge to the physicians due to the non-specificity symptoms as well as the lack of positivity of the subjects for *S. mansoni* eggs in feces in earlier stage of the infection. In this context, abdominal ultrasound can be a complementary tool to assist the diagnoses of the *S. mansoni* infection. The ultrasonographic findings presented in this study were consistent with those described by Barata et al. [11]. According to this report, ultrasonographic evaluation showed non-specific increase in the size of liver, incipient periportal echogenic thickening, in addition to lymph nodes easily identified in the periportal region. The authors have also performed a histological liver analysis from hepatic biopsies of three patients, and the data demonstrated that the periportal thickening seen on ultrasound was probably produced by inflammatory infiltration of the portal tracts caused by schistosomiasis, which disappeared after treatment with oxamniquine.

However, liver biopsy is an invasive procedure that is seldom justified. It is important to mention that the ultrasonographic features of the lymph nodes, liver and spleen in acute schistosomiasis, although highly sensitive, are not pathognomonic of acute schistosomiasis, and are also seen in other infectious diseases such as acute hepatitis and other viral diseases [19, 69, 70].

Normal abdominal lymph nodes are usually not visualized by sonography. Neoplastic lymph nodes are generally rounded and hypoechoic, sometimes with an irregular shape and borders [19, 71, 72]. Lymphomas can also affect periportal and peripancreatic lymph nodes, but there is generally an extensive involvement of other abdominal lymph nodes, mainly retroperitoneal, that is almost anechoic and usually rounded. In this circumstance, the liver and spleen are enlarged and can show focal lesions [19, 72]. Patients with acquired immunodeficiency syndrome (AIDS) can also show hepatoesplenomegaly and abdominal lymphadenopathy, but the echogenicity of the liver is usually increased. Tumors related to AIDS, such as Kaposi's sarcoma, have also been reported as a cause of lymphadenopathy [73]. Mesenteric and periportal lymphadenomegaly is a common finding in blastomycosis and these are almost anechoic [19].

In the current study, we have also evaluated the liver function of acute schistosomiasis patients by the ALT, AST and γ-GT assessment. Comparing with other studies in literature [15, 16], we did not observe changes in any of the enzymes evaluated, suggesting that the hepatocellular function is preserved or minimally compromised in the study population. In patients presenting intestinal or hepatointestinal clinical form of schistosomiasis,it has been observed that the liver function is maintained. In those patients showing the hepatosplenic form, liver function related to protein metabolism was in general changed, but rarely this function is compromised in a broad spectrum. Only after repeated blood spoliation, in the terminal stage of illness, there is strong involvement of the liver parenchymal. According to some authors, when liver cell damage occurs there is an increase of ALT and AST levels, but in the *S. mansoni* infection this type of injury is not commonly observed [74, 75]. On the other hand, the most important cause of increased

γ-GT levels is the chronic stimulation of the microsomal fraction of hepatocytes and the presence of cholestasis [76]. According to Martins & Borges [77], the chronic stimulation of the microsomal occurs only in patients with hepatosplenic form of schistosomiasis. Kardorff et al. [74] observed that the increase of γ-GT occurs only in patients with severe periportal fibrosis, irregular texture liver and collateral vessels.

5. Conclusion

In conclusion, the data presented here suggest that alterations identified by analyses of clinical/laboratorial parameters and ultrasonographic features, although not specific, are compatible with the acute phase of Schistosomiasis mansoni and provide a reliable complementary tool for the diagnosis of the infection.

http://dx.doi.org/10.5772/53047

Acknowledgements

This work was supported by grants from Oswaldo Cruz Foundation (FIOCRUZ), Conselho Nacional de Desenvolvimento Científico e Tecnológico (CNPq), Fundação de Amparo à Pesquisa de Minas Gerais (FAPEMIG), and UNDP World Bank/WHO Special Program for Research and Training in Tropical Diseases. The authors are grateful to the technical staff at the Laboratory of Cellular and Molecular Immunology and the Laboratory of Biomarkers of Diagnosis and Monitoring, Oswaldo Cruz Foundation, Brazil for their invaluable assistance during this study. The authors also thank the Program for Technological Development in Tools for Health - PDTIS - FIOCRUZ for the use of its facilities. OAMF, PMZC, RCO, GG, and ATC are grateful for the CNPq fellowships.

Author details

Matheus Fernandes Costa-Silva**[1,2], Denise da Silveira-Lemos**[1,2,3], Amanda Cardoso de Oliveira Silveira[1], Pedro Henrique Gazzinelli-Guimarães[2], Helena Barbosa Ferraz[1], Cristiano Lara Massara[4], Martin Johannes Enk[5], Maria Carolina Barbosa Álvares[6], Olindo Assis Martins-Filho[1], Paulo Marcos Zech Coelho[5], Rodrigo Corrêa-Oliveira[1,7], Giovanni Gazzinelli[2] and Andréa Teixeira-Carvalho[1,2,7*]

*Address all correspondence to: andreat@cpqrr.fiocruz.br

1 Laboratory of Biomarkers of Diagnosis and Monitoring, Research Center Rene Rachou, FIOCRUZ, Belo Horizonte, MG, Brazil

2 Laboratory of Immunology Cellular and Molecular, Research Center Rene Rachou, FIOC-RUZ, Belo Horizonte, MG, Brazil

3 Laboratory of Immunoparasitology, Department of Biological Science, Institute of Exact Sciences and Biological/NUPEB, Federal University of Ouro Preto, MG, Brasil

4 Laboratory of Helminthology and Medical Malacology, Research Center Rene Rachou, FIOCRUZ, Belo Horizonte, MG, Brazil

5 Laboratory of Schistosomiasis, Research Center Rene Rachou, FIOCRUZ, Belo Horizonte, MG, Brazil

6 Holy House of Mercy of Belo Horizonte, Belo Horizonte, MG, Brazil

7 National Institute of Science and Technology in Tropical Diseases - INCT-DT- Salvador, BA, Brasil

**The authors contributed equally to this study

References

[1] World Health Organization (WHO)First report of joint WHO Expert Committees on the Prevention and Control of Schistosomiasis and Soil-transmitted Helminthiasis. Technical Report Series, Geneva. (2002).

[2] Wilson, M. S, Mentink-kane, M. M, Pesce, J. T, Ramalingam, T. R, Thompson, R, & Wynn, T. A. Immunopathology of schistosomiasis. Immunology Cell Biology (2007). , 85, 148-154.

[3] Passos, A. D, & Amaral, R. S. Esquistossomose mansônica: aspectos epidemiológicos e de controle. Revista da Sociedade Brasileira de Medicina Tropical (1998). , 31, 61-74.

[4] Katz, N, & Peixoto, S. V. Critical analysis of the estimated number of Schistosomiasis mansoni carriers in Brazil. Revista da Sociedade Brasileira de Medicina Tropical (2000). , 33, 303-308.

[5] Raso, P. Esquistossomose mansônica. In: Brasileiro Filho, G. Bogliolo patologia, Rio de Janeiro: Guanabara-Koogan; (2000).

[6] Katz, N. Schistosomiasis control in Brazil. Memórias do Instituto Oswaldo Cruz (1998). , 93, 33-35.

[7] Coura, J. R, & Amaral, R. S. Epidemiological and control aspects of schistosomiasis in Brazilian endemic areas. Memórias do Instituto Oswaldo Cruz (2004). , 99, 13-19.

[8] Amaral, R. S, Tauil, P. L, Lima, D. D, & Engels, D. An analysis of the impact of the Schistosomiasis Control Programme in Brazil. Memórias do Instituto Oswaldo Cruz (2006). , 101, 79-85.

[9] Enk, M. J, Amorim, A, & Schall, V. T. Acute Schistosomiasis Outbreak in the Metropolitan Area of Belo Horizonte, Minas Gerais: Alert about the Risk of Unnoticed Transmission Increased by Growing Rural Tourism. Memórias do Instituto Oswaldo Cruz (2003). , 98, 745-750.

[10] Enk, M. J, Caldeira, R. L, Carvalho, O. S, & Schall, V. T. Rural tourism as risk factor for the transmission of schistosomiasis in Minas Gerais, Brazil. Memórias do Instituto Oswaldo Cruz (2004). , 99, 105-108.

[11] Barata, C. H, Pinto-silva, R. A, & Lambertucci, J. R. Abdominal ultrasound in acute schistosomiasis mansoni. British Journal of Radiology (1999). , 72, 949-952.

[12] Nguyen, L. Q, Estrella, J, Jett, E. A, Grunvald, E. L, Nicholson, L, & Levin, D. L. Acute schistosomiasis in nonimmune travelers: chest CT findings in 10 patients. AJR American Journal Roentgenology (2006). , 186, 1300-1303.

[13] Gazzinelli, G, Lambertucci, J. R, Katz, N, Rocha, R. S, Lima, M. S, & Colley, D. G. Immune responses during human schistosomiasis mansoni: XI. Immunologic status of

patients with acute infections and after treatment. Journal of Immunology (1985). , 135, 2121-2127.

[14] Neves, J. Acute or toxemic form of mansoni's schistosomiasis (Forma aguda ou toxêmica da esquistossomose mansoni). Memórias do Instituto Oswaldo Cruz (1992). , 87, 321-324.

[15] Barbosa, C. S. Montenegro SML, Abath FG, Domingues AL. Specific situations related to acute schistosomiasis in Pernambuco, Brazil. Memórias do Instituto Oswaldo Cruz (2001a). , 96, 169-172.

[16] De Jesus, A. R, Silva, A, Santana, L. B, Magalhães, A, De Jesus, A. A, & Almeida, R. P. Rego MAV, Burattini MN, Pearce EJ, Carvalho EC. Clinical and immunologic evaluation of 31 patients with acute schistosomiasis mansoni. The Journal of Infectious Diseases (2002). , 185, 98-105.

[17] Rabello ALTAcute human schistosomiasis mansoni. Memórias do Instituto Oswaldo Cruz (1995). , 90, 277-280.

[18] Lambertucci, J. R. Da Silva RA, Gerspacher-Lara R, Barata CH. Acute Manson's schistosomiasis: sonographic features. Transactions of the Royal Society of Tropical Medicine and Hygiene (1994). , 88, 76-87.

[19] Rabello ALTPinto-Silva RA, Rocha RS, Katz N. Abominal ultrasonography in acute clinical schistosomiasis mansoni. The American Journal of Tropical Medicine and Hygiene (1994). , 50, 748-752.

[20] Hiatt, R. A, Sotomayor, Z. R, Sanchez, G, Zambrana, M, & Knight, W. B. Factors in the pathogenesis of acute schistosomiasis mansoni. The Journal of Infectious Diseases (1979). , 139, 659-666.

[21] Caldas, I. R, Campi-azevedo, A. C, Oliveira, L. F, Silveira, A. M, Oliveira, R. C, & 25 Gazzinelli, G. Human schistosomiasis mansoni: immune responses during acute and 26 chronic phases of the infection. Acta Tropica (2008)., 108, 109-117.

[22] Oliveira, D. M, Gustavson, S, Silva-teixeira, D. N, & Goes, A. M. Nitric Oxide and IL-10 Production Induced by PIII- A Fraction of Schistosoma mansoni Adult Worm Antigenic Preparation-Associated with Downregulation of In Vitro Granuloma Formation. Human Immunology (1999). , 60, 305-311.

[23] Oliveira, D. M, Silva-teixeira, D. N, Carmo, S. A, & Goes, A. M. Role of nitric oxide on human schistosomiasis mansoni: up-regulation of in vitro granuloma formation by L-NAME. Nitric Oxide (1998). , 2, 57-62.

[24] Skinner, H. A, Holt, S, Schuller, R, Roy, J, & Israel, Y. Identification of alcohol abuse using laboratory markers and a history of trauma. Annals of Internal Medicine (1984). , 101, 847-51.

[25] Stoltzfus, R. J, & Dreyfuss, M. L. Guidelines for the use of iron supplements to prevent and treat iron deficiency anemia. International Nutritional Anemia Consultative Group, Washington: (1998).

[26] Katz, N, Chaves, A, & Pellegrino, J. A simple device for quantitative stool thick smear technique in schistosomiasis mansoni. Revista do Instituto de Medicina Tropical de São Paulo (1972)., 14, 397-400.

[27] Abdel-wahab, M. F, Esmat, G, Farrag, A, Boraey, Y. A, & Strickland, G. T. Grading of hepatic schistosomiasis by the use of ultrasonography. The American Journal of Tropical Medicine and Hygiene (1992)., 46, 403-408.

[28] Homeida, M, Abdel-gadir, A. F, Cheever, A. W, & Bennett, J. L. Arbah BMO, Ibrahim SZ, Abdel-Salam IM, Dafalla AA, Nash T. Diagnosis of pathologically confirmed Symmers' periportal fibrosis by ultrasonography: A prospective blinded study. The American Journal of Tropical Medicine and Hygiene (1988)., 38, 86-91.

[29] Cerri, G. G, Alves, V. A, & Magalhães, A. Hepatosplenic schistosomiasis mansoni: ultrasound manifestations. Radiology (1984)., 153, 777-780.

[30] Barbosa, C. S. Domingues ALC, Abath F, Montenegro SML, Guida U, Carneiro J, Tobosa B, Moraes CNL, Spinelli. Epidemiologia da esquistossomose aguda na praia de Porto de Galinhas, Pernambuco, Brasil. Caderno de Saúde Pública (2001b). , 17, 725-8.

[31] Barbosa, C. S, & Barbosa, F. S. Padrão epidemiológico da esquistossomose em comunidade de pequenos produtores rurais de Pernambuco. Caderno de Saúde Pública (1998)., 14, 129-137.

[32] Suassuna, A, & Coura, J. R. Esquistossomose mansoni no Estado da Guanabara: Aspectos epidemiológicos relacionados as migrações internas. Revista da Sociedade Brasileira de Medicina Tropical (1969)., 2, 59-71.

[33] Sturrock, R. F. Schistosomiasis epidemiology and control: how did we get here and where should we go? Memórias do Instituto Oswaldo Cruz (2001)., 96, 17-27.

[34] Ferreira, L. F, Naveira, J. B, & Silva, J. R. Fase toxêmica da esquistossomose mansoni. Revista do Instituto de Medicina Tropical de São Paulo (1960)., 2, 112-120.

[35] Ferreira, H, Oliveira, C. A, Bittencourt, D, & Katz, N. Carneiro LFC, Grinbaum E, Veloso C, Dias RP, Alvarenga RJ, Dias CB. A fase aguda da esquistossomose mansoni. Jornal Brasileiro de Medicina (1966)., 11, 54-67.

[36] Massara, C. L, Amaral, G. L, Caldeira, R. L, Drummond, S. C, Enk, M. J, & Carvalho, O. S. Schistosomiasis in an ecotourism area in Minas Gerais State, Brazil. Caderno de Saúde Pública (2008)., 24(7), 1709-1712.

[37] Lunde, M. N, & Ottesen, E. A. Enzyme-linked immunosorbent assay (ELISA) for detecting IgM and IgE antibodies in human schistosomiasis. The American Journal of Tropical Medicine and Hygiene (1980). , 29, 82-85.

[38] Evengard, B, & Hammarstrom, L. Smith CIE, Linder E. Early antibody responses in human schistosomiasis. Clinical & Experimental Immunology (1990). , 80, 69-76.

[39] Pessoa, S. B, & Amorin, J. P. Notas sobre a epidemiologia da esquistossomose mansônica em algumas localidades de Alagoas. Revista Brasileira de Medicina (1957). , 14, 420-422.

[40] Kloetzel, K. Schistosomiasis in Brazil: does social development suffice? Parasitology Today (1989). , 5, 386-391.

[41] Lambertucci, J. R. Acute schistosomiasis: Clinical, diagnostic and therapeutic features. Revista do Instituto de Medicina Tropical de São Paulo (1993). , 35, 399-404.

[42] Garcia-palmieri, M. R, & Marcial-rojas, R. A. The protein manifestations of schistosomiasis mansoni. Annals of Internal Medicine (1962). , 57, 763-775.

[43] Rocha MOCPedroso ERP, Greco DB, Lambertucci JR, Katz N, Rocha RL, Rocha RS, Rezende DF, Neves J. Pathogenetic factors of acute schistosomiasis mansoni: correlation of worm burden, IgE, blood eosinophilia and intensity of clinical manifestations. Tropical Medicine & International Health (1996). , 2, 213-220.

[44] Diaz-rivera, R. S, Ramos-morales, F, & Koppisch, E. Acute Manson's schistosomiasis. The American Journal of Medicine (1956). , 21, 918-943.

[45] Greco, D. B, Pedroso, E. R, Lambertucci, J. R, Rocha, M. O, Coelho, P. M, Raso, P, & Ferreira, C. S. Pulmonary involvement in schistosomiasis mansoni. Memórias do lnstituto Oswaldo Cruz (1987). , 82, 221-227.

[46] Neves, J. Esquistossomose Mansoni: Clínica da Forma Aguda ou Toxêmica. Rio de Janeiro: Medsi Médico e Clínica Ltda (1986).

[47] Rocha MOCPedroso ERP, Neves J, Rocha RS, Greco DB, Lambertucci JR, Rocha RL, Katz N. Characterization of the non-apparent clinical form in the initial phase of schistosomiasis mansoni. Revista do lnstituto de Medicina Tropical de São Paulo (1993). , 35, 247-251.

[48] Babapulle, F. B. The eosinophilias, including the idiopathic hypereosinophilic syndrome. British Journal of Haematology (2003). , 121, 203-223.

[49] Rumbley, C. A, Sugaya, H, Zekavat, S. A, El Refaei, M, Perrin, P. J, & Phillips, S. M. Activated eosinophils are the major source of Th2-associated cytokines in the schistosome granuloma. Journal Immunology (1999). , 162, 1003-1009.

[50] De Andres, B, Rakasz, E, Hagen, M, Mccormik, M. L, Mueller, A. L, Elliot, D, Metwali, A, Sandor, M, Britigan, B. E, Weinstock, J. V, & Lynch, R. G. Lack of Fc-epsilon re-

ceptors on murine eosinophils: implications for the functional significance of elevated IgE and eosinophils in parasitic infections. Blood (1997). , 89, 3826-36.

[51] Cara, D. C, Negrao-correa, D, & Teixeira, M. M. Mechanisms underlying eosinophil trafficking and their relevance in vivo. Histology and Histopathology (2000). , 15, 899-920.

[52] Gleich, G. J, Loegering, D. A, & Maldonado, J. E. Identification of a major basic protein in guinea pig eosinophil granules. The Journal of Experimental Medicine (1973). , 137, 1459-1461.

[53] Weller, P. F. The immunology of eosinophils. The New England Journal of Medicine (1991). , 324, 1110-1118.

[54] Gleich, G. J, Frigas, E, Loegering, D. A, Wassom, D. L, & Steinmuller, D. Cytotoxic properties of the eosinophil major basic protein. Journal of Immunology (1979). , 123, 2925-2927.

[55] Butterworth, A. E, Wassom, D. L, Gleich, G. J, Loegering, D. A, & David, J. R. Damage to schistosomula of Schistosoma mansoni induced by eosinophil major basic protein. Journal of Immunology (1979). , 122, 221-229.

[56] Jong, E. C. Mahmoud AAF, Klebanoff SJ. Peroxidase-mediated toxicity to schistosomula of Schistosoma mansoni. Journal of lmmunology (1981). , 126, 468-477.

[57] Ackerman, S. J, Gleich, G. J, Loegering, D. A, Richardson, B. A, & Butterworth, A. E. Comparative toxicity of purified human eosinophil granule cationic proteins for schistosomula of Schistosoma mansoni. The American Journal of Tropical Medicine and Hygiene (1985). , 34, 735-745.

[58] Gleich, G. J, Schroeter, A. L, Marcoux, J. P, Sachs, M. I, Connell, O, & Kohler, E. J. PF. Episodic angiodema associated with eosinophilia. The New England Journal of Medicine (1984). , 310, 1621-1626.

[59] De Souza, J. R. Morais CNL, Aroucha ML, Miranda PJC, Barbosa CS, Domingues ALC, Junior LBC, Abath FGC, Montenegro SML. Treatment of human acute schistosomiasis with oxamniquine induces an increase in interferon-γ response to Schistosoma mansoni antigens. Memórias do Instituto Oswaldo Cruz (2007). , 102(2), 225-228.

[60] Pereira, W. R, Kloos, H, Crawford, S. B, Velásquez-melendez, J. G, Matoso, L. F, Fujiwara, R. T, Cançado, G. G, Loverde, P. T, Correa-oliveira, R, & Gazzinelli, A. Schistosoma mansoni infection in a rural area of the Jequitinhonha Valley, Minas Gerais, Brazil: analysis of exposure risk. Acta Tropica (2010). , 113(1), 34-41.

[61] Oliveira, D. M, Gustavson, S, Silva-teixeira, D. N, & Goes, A. M. Nitric Oxide and IL-10 Production Induced by PIII- A Fraction of Schistosoma mansoni Adult Worm Antigenic Preparation-Associated with Downregulation of In Vitro Granuloma Formation. Human Immunology (1999). , 60, 305-311.

[62] Brunet, L. R. Nitric oxide in parasitic infections. International Immunopharmacology (2001)., 1, 1457-1467.

[63] Colasanti, M, Gradoni, L, Mattu, M, Persichini, T, Salvati, L, Venturini, G, & Ascenzi, P. Molecular basis for the anti-parasitic effect on NO. International Journal of Molecular Medicine (2002)., 9, 131-134.

[64] Rai, G, Sayed, A. A, Lea, W. A, Luecke, H. F, Chakrapani, H, Prast-nielsen, S, Jadhav, A, Leister, W, Shen, M, Inglese, J, Austin, C. P, Keefer, L, Arnér, E. S, Simeonov, A, Maloney, D. J, Williams, D. L, & Thomas, C. J. Structure mechanism insights and the role of nitric oxide donation guide the development of oxadiazole-2-oxides as therapeutic agents against schistosomiasis. Journal of Medicinal Chemistry (2009). , 52, 6474-83.

[65] James, S. L, & Glaven, J. Macrophage cytotoxicity against schistosomula of Schistosoma mansoni involves arginine-dependent production of reactive nitrogen intermediates. Journal of Immunology (1989)., 143, 4208-4212.

[66] Brunet, L. R, Beall, M, Dunne, D. W, & Pearce, E. J. Nitric oxide and the th2 response combine to prevent severe hepatic damage during Schistosoma mansoni infection. Journal of Immunology (1999)., 163, 4976-4977.

[67] Abath FGCMorais CNL, Montenegro CEL, Wynn TA, Montenegro SML. Immunopathogrnic mechanisms in schistosomiasis: what can be learnt from human studies? Trends in Parasitology (2006)., 2, 85-91.

[68] Ramos, R. P, Costa, V. M, Melo, C. F, Souza, V. M, Malagueño, E, Coutinho, E. M, Abath, F. G, & Montenegro, S. M. Preliminary results on interleukin-4 and interleukin-10 cytokine production in malnourished, inducible nitric oxide synthase-deficient mice with schistosomiasis mansoni infection. Memórias do Instituto Oswaldo Cruz (2006)., 101(1), 331-332.

[69] Forsberg, L, Floren, C. M, Mederstrom, E, & Prytz, H. Ultrasound examination in diffuse liver disease: clinical significance of enlarged lymph nodes in the hepato-duodenal ligament. Acta Radiologica (1987)., 28, 281-284.

[70] Giorgio, A, Amoroso, P, Lettien, G, Firelli, L, De Stefano, G, Pesce, G, Scala, V, & Pierri, P. Ultrasound evaluation of uncomplicated and complicated acute viral hepatitis. Journal of Clinical Ultrasound (1986)., 14, 675-679.

[71] Marchal, G, Oyen, R, Verschakelen, J, Gelin, J, Baert, A. L, & Stessens, R. C. Sonographic appearence of normal lymph nodes. American Institute of Ultrasound in Medicine (1985)., 4, 417-419.

[72] Vassallo, P, Wernecke, K, Roos, N, & Peters, P. E. Differentiation of benign from malignant superficial lymphadenopathy: the role of high-resolution US. Radiology (1992)., 183, 215-220.

[73] Yee, J. M, Raghavendra, B. N, Horii, S. C, & Ambrosino, M. Abdominal sonography in AIDS. A review. American Institute of Ultrasound in Medicine (1993). , 12, 705-714.

[74] Kardorff, R, Gabone, R. M, Mugashe, C, Obiga, D, Ramarokoto, C. E, Mahlert, C, Spannbrucker, N, Lang, A, Günzler, V, & Gryseels, B. Ehrich JHH, Doehring E. Schistosoma mansoni-related morbidity on Ukerewe Island, Tanzania: clinical, ultrasonographical and biochemical parameters. Tropical Medicine & International Health (1997). , 2, 230-239.

[75] Aquino RTRChieffi PP, Catunda SM, Araújo MF, Ribeiro MCSA, Taddeo EF, Rolim EG. Hepatitis B and C virus markers among patients with hepatosplenic mansonic schistosomiasis. Revista do Instituto de Medicina Tropical de São Paulo (2000). , 42, 313-320.

[76] Alves-júnior, A, Fontes, D. A, & Melo, V. A. Machado MCC, Cruz JF, Santos EAS. Hipertensão portal esquistossomótica: influência do fluxo sanguíneo portal nos níveis séricos das enzimas hepáticas. Arquivos de Gastroenterologia (2003). , 40, 203-208.

[77] Martins, R. D, & Borges, D. R. Ethanol challenge in non-alcoholic patients with schistosomiasis. Journal of Clinical Pathology (1993). , 46, 250-253.

Chapter 6

Spinal Cord Schistosomiasis

André Ricardo Ribas Freitas and
Rodrigo Nogueira Angerami

Additional information is available at the end of the chapter

http://dx.doi.org/10.5772/53771

1. Introduction

The human central nervous system (CNS) may be affected by infections of several species in the *Schistosoma* genus that infect men. One of the CNS clinical presentation is the spinal cord schistosomiasis, a potentially severe disease, yet, for a long time, a poorly recognized clinical presentation of Schistosomiasis. However, recently, probably as a consequence significant improvements in diagnostic methods, more attention is being given to this clinical form of Schistosomiasis. This emerging medical and scientific interest about the spinal cord schistosomiasis has allowed a better comprehension of its clinical impact and importance as a previously unrecognized public health problem.

Schistosomiasis is among the parasitic diseases with the highest epidemiological importance in the world. According to the World Health Organization, schistosomiasis occurs in 76 countries and 230 million individuals require treatment annually [1,2]. Of these, about 100 million present some clinical manifestation and 20 million present severe forms of the disease [1-5]. Annually, over 200.000 people die as a consequence of schistosomiasis. In the year 2010, around 33.5 million people were treated. Despite advances in the control of the disease, with lowering of mortality and morbidity, schistosomiasis still represents a challenge to public health and has increased its area of transmission throughout the years [2]. Since it hits the poorer regions of the world, being associated with precarious sanitary and adverse social-economical conditions, this disease has been neglected. With the increase of migratory flow and adventure tourism travels, innumerable schistosomiasis cases have been occurring, even in non-endemic countries [6-13]. Schistosomiasis is a disease caused by trematode worms, belonging to the Schistosoma genus. There are many species which affect man in different clinical manifestations, elimination methods, intermediary hosts and geographical distribution. These species share the same pattern in reproductive cycle, the transmission occurring through eggs, a proportion of which are eliminated through urine (*S. haematobium*) or feces (*S. mansoni*, *S. japonicum* and others). These eggs release larvae (miracidium) that infect freshwater molluscs in which the parasites multiply through asexual reproduction. These molluscs release aquatic larvae (cercariae) that actively penetrate the skin of a new, vertebrate host. These larvae become adults that inhabit inside the veins in the digestive system (*S. mansoni* and *S. japonicum*) and of the urinary system (*S. haematobium*). The geographic distribution of each species is varied and depends on the presence of molluscs capable of serving as hosts (each *Schistosoma* species has different molluscs as hosts). Precarious sanitary conditions also contribute in the definition of locations where schistosomiasis occurs [14]. *Schistosoma mansoni* occurs in 74 countries located in Africa, the Middle East, South America and the Caribbean. Its eggs measure about 60 x 140 μm, with lateral spine and are eliminated in the feces, being a main cause of intestinal, hepatosplenic, cardiopulmonary and cerebral diseases, aside from being the main cause of spinal cord schistosomiasis. *S. haematobium* occurs in Africa and in the Middle East and its eggs measure about 60 x 150 μm, with terminal spine, are eliminated in the urine and on rare occasions in the feces, being the mains cause of urinary diseases and spinal cord schistosomiasis. *S. japonicum*, *S. mekongi* and *S. malayensis* occur in Asia (they are also called *S. japonicum*-like); eggs measure about 60 x 100 μm, lack spine and are eliminated in the feces, causing hepatic diseases, cerebral neuroschistosomiasis, although there have been rare reports of cases in which spinal cord schistosomiasis was caused by *S. japonicum*. S. intercalatum occurs in Africa. Eggs are eliminated in the feces. It causes mild intestinal disease but not neuroschistosomiasis, being the least important species, clinically. The presence of spines in the eggs of *S. mansoni* and *S. haematobium* might explain why medullar and cerebral neuroschistosomiasis are more common in these species. Spine makes it more difficult for the eggs to travel through the vertebral veins, causing them to be stuck in the lumbar or thoracic spinal cord. *S. japonium*'s eggs, being smaller and lacking spine, migrate more easily to the brain through these veins, crossing the spinal cord without sticking to it. There are, still, species belonging to the *Schistosomatidae* family (ex: Trichobilharzia regenti) that can cause cercarial dermatitis (or *summer's itch*) without, however, reaching adult life in men and, therefore, not having any major clinical importance.

2. Clinical forms of schistosomiasis

2.1. Acute phase

Acute forms are basically cercarial dermatitis or summer's itch, cutaneous lesion secondary to the penetration of the skin by the cercaria, and Katayama's fever (or syndrome), which is also called acute or toxemic schistosomiasis and occurs, in genera, after three to nine weeks of cercariae penetration, when they have already become adult worms and start laying eggs. Toxemia is secondary to hypersensitivity reactions to the parasite, being characteristic to patients who do not reside in endemic areas and that are exposed to contaminated water bodies [15,16]. This form presents with fever, chills, cough, weakness, weight loss, diarrhea, vomiting, urticarial reactions, hepatosplenomegaly and eosinophilia. These manifestations last, in general, a few days but can last months and, in rare cases, be fatal. These patients present big periovular necrotic-exudative granulomas dispersed throughout the intestines, liver and other organs [17], and generally present spontaneous clinical improvement after a few weeks, but treatment associating schistosomicides and corticosteroids reduce the persistence time of symptoms and prevents evolution into the chronic phase.

Species	Regions where it occurs	Main affected organs	Most common neurological forms
S. mansoni	Sub-Saharan Africa, Brazil, Egypt, Middle-East, other regions in Africa and in the Americas	Liver, spleen and intestines	Spinal cord schistosomiasis (mainly) and cerebral schistosomiasis
S. haematobium	Sub-Saharan Africa, Brazil, Egypt, Middle-East, other regions in Africa	Bladder, urethra and ureter	Spinal cord (mainly) and cerebral schistosomiasis
S. japonicum and *S. japonicum*-like	China, South-East Asia and Pacific islands	Liver, spleen and intestines	Cerebral schistosomiasis (mainly) and spinal cord schistosomiasis

Table 1. Geographic distribution, usually affected organs, and most frequent neurological forms according *Schistosoma* species

2.2. Chronic phase

Schistosomiasis' chronic phase is frequently asymptomatic. Symptoms occur with more frequency in patients who are repeatedly exposed to transmissions focuses and end up developing high worm burden. Chronic forms depend on the involved species. Schistosomiasis mansoni chronic forms are usually classified as: intestinal, hepatointestinal, hepatosplenic and decompensated hepatosplenic. In the intestinal and hepatosplenic forms patients usually do not present significant symptoms, but when present they may include abdominal discomfort, fecal urgency, episodes of diarrhea with eventual mucus or blood. Hepatic lesions are caused by egg embolism secondary to inflammatory reaction, but without significant clinical repercussions. With progression of infection and chronic inflammatory process, these patients may present significant periportal fibrosis, leading to portal hypertension. This phase is called hepatosplenic and the patient may suffer ascites and severe esophageal varices [17]. Schistosomiasis japonica may cause the same kinds of manifestations, although liver function is usually more compromised. In schistosomiasis haematobia, oviposition may cause bladder inflammation, alongside blood in the urine and urinary urgency. Lesions in the urinary tract may cause fibrosis and urinary obstruction, leading to obstructive uropathy and increasing the risk of bladder cancer. These chronic forms depend fundamentally on high worm burdens, therefore they are diseases that affect mainly inhabitants of endemic areas. For instance, hepatosplenic forms of schistosomiasis mansoni are more frequent in areas with high endemicity and very rare in areas of low endemicity. Differently, ectopic forms of schistosomiasis occur as consequence of egg or work accumulation in any organ of the patient and, therefore, is not related to high worm burdens. Thus, it can occur in patients of endemic areas or in patients of non-endemic areas with casual exposure to the focus of transmission.

3. Spinal cord schistosomiasis

The human central nervous system (CNS) may be affected by infections of several species in the *Schistosoma* genus that infect men, excluding S. intercalatum. Curiously, other species of Schistosomatidae, such as *Trichobilharzia regenti*, may cause brain or medullar lesions in water birds, but in man causes only swimmer's itch [18-20]. The first human case of neurological lesion cause by *Schistosoma* was described in 1889 by Yamagiwa in the necropsy of a patient with epilepsy that presented cerebral granulomas. It is curious that *S. japonicum* life cycle was described 15 years later, a fact that allowed the *a posteriori* identification of the eggs present in those granulomas [21,22]. In 1905, Shimamura and Tsunoda demonstrated for the first time the presence of *S. japonicum* in the spinal cord of a patient with transverse myelitis. Despite the fact that *S. japonicum* was the first species described as a cause of spinal cord medullar lesion, this species has been the less frequently associated with such lesions in the Schistosoma genera. The first case of medullar lesion caused by *S. mansoni* was described in 1930 by Muller and Stender and found in a 26 year old patient who had been to Brazil. In 1948, Faust published a review on the 82 cases of ectopic schistosomiasis described thus far [23]. Among these, there were 56 patients with brain compromising and 8 with medullar lesions in the spinal cord. In that occasion, the author highlighted the importance of this form of disease, given that the number of cases was not inconsiderable and that the consequences were, in general, devastating. "In reports of the cases, it has been customary that most authors address ectopic schistosomiasis as rare or really rare. These designations are no more applicable, despite these syndromes being relatively infrequent" [23]. In the same year, Kane and Most wrote yet another review article on literature concerning neurological lesions caused by *Schistosoma*, including the medullary and brain forms, and called attention to the occurrence of 25 cases of cerebral neuroschistosomiasis japonica among north-American soldiers in the Second World War, between the years of 1944 and 1946 [24]. In this study, 88% (22 cases) of the initial fecal exams of North-American military patients with cerebral neuroschistosomiasis japonica were negative for eggs in the stool samples in the first examination and that 40% (10 cases) remained negative after several serial examinations. All patients had confirmation of *Schistosoma* eggs in pathological anatomy examinations, obtained through CNS biopsy or necropsy. The author, at the time, already said that "Cautious and repeated fecal examinations are important for clinical diagnosis, but specific treatment must not be postponed if there are adequate evidence for presumptive diagnosis, even because all fecal examinations may be negative for eggs even when the patient already shows neurological symptoms". Despite the fact that the authors were referring to cerebral neuroschistosomiasis japonica, the same advice is valid for spinal cord schistosomiasis today.

Up until the 1980's, medullar lesion caused by *Schistosoma* was, in most published cases, confirmed through fragments of nervous tissue obtained through biopsy or necropsy. In 1985, Scrimgeour and Gedjusek published a scientific literature review of the years between 1930 and 1984 in which they identified 52 cases of spinal cord schistosomiasis mansoni and 12 cases of spinal cord schistosomiasis haematobia, confirmed by pathological anatomy medullar examinations. On the occasion, the authors highlighted the importance of suspecting neuroschistosomiasis in any patient who had been exposed to the risk of infection and presented neurological manifestations [25]. The authors reaffirmed that the patients in general had no previous manifestation of schistosomiasis and that only 22% of *S. mansoni* carriers had eggs found in their feces or rectum biopsy and only 25% of the *S. haematobium* carriers had eggs found in their urine or feces [25]. This difficulty in finding the eggs is not casual, nor an abnormal occurrence. It is part of the disease's laboratory findings pattern [26]. Despite having already done some serological examinations that could have confirmed infection by the parasites even without finding eggs, the diagnosis of spinal cord schistosomiasis was still very complicated and controversial at that time, specially because there were no detailed imaging examinations. Some studies already used presumptive diagnosis criteria, in which the presence of lower thoracic or high lumbar medullar symptoms, the demonstration of exposure to *Schistosoma* through parasitological or immunological methods, and the exclusion of other causes for myelitis were enough for attributing the clinical manifestation to spinal cord schistosomiasis [27]. There were, still, some divergences in the literature regarding the acceptance of the parasitological e/or immunological methods for case confirmation, but the risk of sequelae involved in biopsying the medulla led to the confirmation of the diagnosis through pathological anatomical methods being abandoned [28-31]. In the last decades, spinal cord schistosomiasis diagnosis has been reached through confirmation of *Schistosoma* infection using pararitological or serological methods associated with the exclusion of other causes for myelopathy [32-37].

With the technological improvement in the field of immunological methods and imaging examinations, including the introduction of Computerized Tomography (CT) and, mainly, Magnetic Resonance Imaging (MRI), differential diagnosis with other causes of myelopathy has become easier. This can explain, at least in part, the great amount of articles being published in this area [22,38-44]. With the increase in interest for adventure tourism, a growing number of spinal cord schistosomiasis cases, who live in non-endemic areas and are infected in their leisure time, have been described in the literature. Spinal cord schistosomiasis, which had been considered a rare disease from the beginning of the 20th century to the early 80's, now appeared to have been, in fact, under-recognized. In the last years, it has attracted more and more the interest of researchers and is considered one of the forms of schistosomiasis that must be reevaluated from the point of view of disease burden by Public Health Organizations [45].

There are, in the literature, studies that allow an evaluation on the incidence or prevalence in the population with schistosomiasis or exposed to the risk of schistosomiasis. In bibliographical studies of international literature between 1930 and 1984, 64 patients were identified (12 with *S. haematobium* and 52 with *S. mansoni*) and described in the literature [25]. Another bibliographical study published, which included 12 years worth of publications, identified 280 patients with described in the literature [21]. This sudden increase in the number of publications regarding this disease reiterates the hypotheses that the improvement in diagnostic methods has allowed an increase in the recognition of this disease. Thus, neuroschistosomiasis must now be recognized as a problem to be considered by the developers of public policies.

The proportion of patients who go from schistosomiasis to spinal cord schistosomiasis is unknown. But a study done in Bahia with 212 patients with non-traumatic medullar lesion shows that 9.9% (21 cases) of patients had schistosomotic etiology [30]. In another, similar study performed at the Sarah Kubitschek Hospital, in Brazil, with 231 patients, this etiology corresponded to close to 6% of the patients (13 cases) of non-traumatic medullar lesion seen in 4.5 years [36]. There are several indications that this disease has been under-diagnosed [46-49] in endemic areas because of the difficulty of access to more sophisticated diagnostic methods and, in more developed areas, because of the lack of knowledge on the part of the doctors about this disease [26]. This situation has been changing in the last years, particularly in Brazil, due to the improvement in diagnostic tools and better access to medical attention in the country. This may explain the increase of cases in patients of this country that are reported in the literature.

Knowledge of the epidemiological profile of the patient with spinal cord schistosomiasis can be obtained based on case reports or serial cases [26, 42, 50-52]. Spinal cord schistosomiasis occurs more frequently in male patients, with ages between 15 and 50, having low worm burden, up until then not presenting symptomatic neuroschistosomiasis, presenting intestinal and hepatointestinal forms, living in non-endemic areas (who had an eventual exposure to risk of infection) or in endemic areas.

There are several indications that a greater risk for spinal cord schistosomiasis cases in patients is present for patients with low worm burdens [53-55]. This means that spinal cord schistosomiasis can occur in patients with low risk for severe hepatosplenic forms. They are patients who do not present symptoms relating to the digestive tract, which often may lead the assisting physician not to think of schistosomiasis diagnosis. Other patients, aside from not having digestive symptoms, are not frequently exposed to the risk of transmission, making the diagnosis even harder. Examples of said patient profile are tourists who have been only sporadically exposed in areas of schistosomiasis transmission [27, 56, 57], patients who live in urban areas who, usually, have sporadic contact with transmission focuses [58], residents of areas that are recent focuses of transmission [56], and residents of areas with low prevalence for schistosomiasis [26].

Despite the severity of sequelae and disabilities caused by spinal cord schistosomiasis, this form of schistosomiasis is still not being considered in the development of public policies that aim to control the morbidity of schistosomiasis [1, 45, 58].

4. Physiopathology

Knowledge on spinal cord schistosomiasis physiopathology has greatly improved in the last years, although some blanks still remain. It is known that periovular granulomas play a central role in medullar lesion [54, 55]. Although signs of vasculitis with immune complexes deposits close to the granulomas can be found [59], it is believed that these findings have a secondary role in the lesion. The mass effect produced by the granuloma and the edema that surrounds it may lead to the compression of internal structures to the spinal canal, causing secondary and definitive ischemic lesions. The eggs get to the medulla via the Batson venus plexus through embolization or through anomalous worm migration, in which case they would lay their eggs next to the medulla [54, 55]. This plexus was first described in 1940 by Batson, who intended to explain a mechanism for metastases being dispersed to the CNS [60]. It is a network of valveless veins that connects the inferior vena cava to the veins in the vertebrae. This plexus allows the embolization of eggs without the need for collateral circulation or arteriovenous shunts, seen only in the hepatosplenic and cardiopulmonary forms of schistosomiasis. The eggs of *S. mansoni* and of S. *haematobium* are larger, oval-shaped and have spine (terminal in *S. haematobium* and lateral in *S. mansoni*), which may explain why these species are associated with different neurological manifestations, most of them attributed to lesions in the lower levels segments of spinal cord, and, less frequently, higher manifestations in the spinal cord's medulla [54]. *S. japonicum* eggs are smaller, lack a spine, and are round, allowing them to reach the brain more easily through these anastomoses, causing a smaller proportion of medullar lesions. The probability of these eggs getting to the places where the lesion occurred through ectopic oviposition is reinforced in some situations, in which several eggs are found very close together, or even creating cordons. Aside from that, worm couples were found near these locations in medullar veins. The highest proportion of causes occurring in man can be explained by their greater exposure to focuses of transmission and by differences in pelvic anatomy between both sexes [54].

The greater proportion of spinal cord schistosomiasis cases in patients who present the initial form of schistosomiasis when compared to the ones who present the advanced form appears to have immunological and hemodynamic reasons. Pittella and Lana-Peixoto studied extensively the occurrence of *Schistosoma* eggs in necropsy nervous tissue samples, and found eggs in 26% of the patients who presented hepatosplenic forms and 61,1% of the patients who presented cardiopulmonary forms [53, 61]. Periovular reactions in the CNS are intense in patients presenting medullary forms of neuroschistosomiasis, with periovular necrotic-exudative granulomas that are typically found in the initial stages of the disease (Figures 1 and 2).

Patients with hepatosplenic and cardiopulmonary forms usually present discreet periovular reaction, without granulomatous response or with smaller granulomas, in non-productive stages and located in several regions of the CNS [53-55, 61, 62]. Only 10% of the patients who had eggs in the CNS in the necropsy, and presented these advanced forms also presented neurological symptoms when alive. [53]. One of the suggested mechanisms to explain egg dispersion in cases of patients with hepatosplenic and cardiopulmonary schistosomiasis is that the eggs would get to the CNS by bypassing through collateral portal-like circulation and intrapulmonary arteriovenous shunting, secondary to hemodynamic alterations common to these advanced forms of schistosomiasis. In these cases there is major egg dispersion through the CNS through anastomoses, but few of these eggs cause symptoms given that the inflammatory response in these patients is usually discreet. In patients presenting schistosomiasis in the intestinal and hepatointestinal forms, the most viable way for the worm couples to reach the CNS is Batson's plexus and, therefore, the most common neurological forms are medullary.

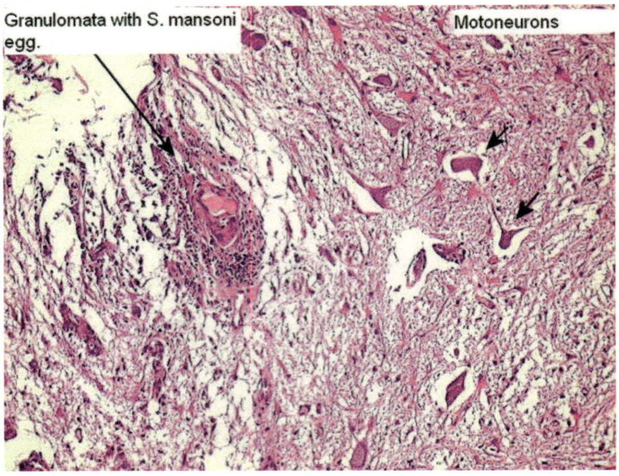

Figure 1. Periovular reaction with granuloma in spinal cord biopsy fragment of a patient with neuroschistosomiasis caused by *Schistosoma mansoni* infection (Optical microscopy, hematoxiline eosine method).

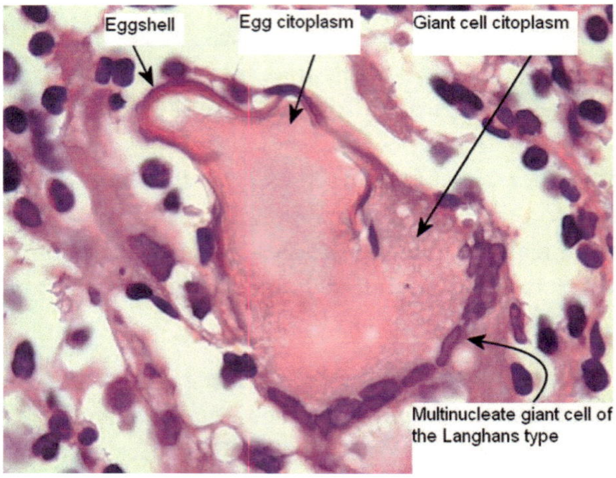

Figure 2. Periovular reaction with granulomatous response in spinal cord biopsy fragment of a patient with neuroschistosomiasis caused by *Schistosoma mansoni* infection (Optical microscopy, hematoxiline eosine method).

5. Schistosomiasis and immune response

During the disease's evolution, immune responses change over time, there being several cytokines that participate with different responses at each moment. Immediately after infection by *Schistosoma*, there is a predominance of T-helper (Th) lymphocytes in action, producing interferon gamma (INF-γ), interleukin (IL)-2, and tumor necrosis factor (TNF)-α. This stage usually lasts an average of 5 to 6 weeks in murine models that corresponds to the acute phase of the disease (Katayama Fever) in humans [63-65]. With the evolution of the disease, this response is substituted by Th2 type and its associated cytokines are IL-4, IL-5, IL-10 and IL-13. At this stage, it is more common for spinal cord schistosomiasis to happen, as shown by the elevated concentration of these cytokines not only in the CSF, but also in the blood and serum from patients with spinal cord schistosomiasis [66]. Concentration of TH1 type cytokines found in patients with spinal cord schistosomiasis was also lower than in patients from the control group. In other words, spinal cord schistosomiasis seems to be more common in patients who present TH2 type of immunological responses, corresponding to the initial chronic phase of the patient with schistosomiasis, right after the acute phase of the disease, but that may last for years. CD4+ T-cells (T-helper) play a central role in the formation of the granuloma, so much so that in rats without a thymus there is no formation of granulomas and patients with CD4+ T-cell depletion granulomas that may form are, generally, smaller [63-65].

With the evolution of schistosomiasis, TH2 polarized response is attenuated by suppressor T-cells, which modulate immune response, diminishing the production of cytokines, inhibiting the formation of granulomas, and diminishing the size of the granulomas that do form [63-65], a situation which has been observed in patients with hepatosplenic and cardiopulmonary schistosomiasis. This may explain the reason why there are many patients with advanced forms who present multiple eggs in the CNS, without inflammatory reaction around them and that, therefore, do not elicit any symptom [54, 55, 66].

6. Clinical manifestations

The typical clinical manifestations of spinal cord spinal cord schistosomiasis is acute or subacute and presents with lumbar pain with or without radiation to lower limbs, evolving with diminishing of muscular strength in these limbs, with the possibility of presenting, in addition, sensory alterations such as hypoaesthesia, paresthesia and dysesthesia [26]. Clinically, there may be myeloradicular or radicular compromising of the medulla, with lesions in several segments of the medulla. Lesions which are higher in the spinal cord and in a functional section of the medulla may present signs of pyramidal liberation, such as Babinski's or hyperreflexia in the lower limbs. Lower lesions may present themselves as cauda equina syndrome with hypo- or areflexia in the lower limbs and unresponsive plantar-cutaneous reflex. Patients with spinal cord schistosomiasis usually present fecal and urinary retention, or other sphincter alterations, aside from erectile dysfunction [26]. The amount of time between the beginning of the symptoms and the establishment of the complete manifestation normally ranges from a few days to a couple of weeks [21, 26, 66-68]. In general, these patients do no present systemic symptoms. Some patients may present cephalalgia, vomiting and other signs of meningeal irritation, such as Kernig's, Brudzinski's or nuchal rigidity [67]. When there is radiculopathy, patient may present Lasègue's sign. Spinal cord schistosomiasis' typical triad is diminishing of muscular strength, with sensory alterations in the lower limbs associated with bladder dysfunction, this triad is found in 92,6% of the cases [26].

7. Diagnosis

Spinal cord schistosomiasis' diagnosis it not always simple, but there is a consensus that an adequate diagnosis must include typical clinical manifestation (medullar and/or radicular symptoms), proof of exposure to *Schistosoma* through parasitological or immunological methods, and exclusion of other possible causes of myelopathy [26, 27, 32-37, 67-69].

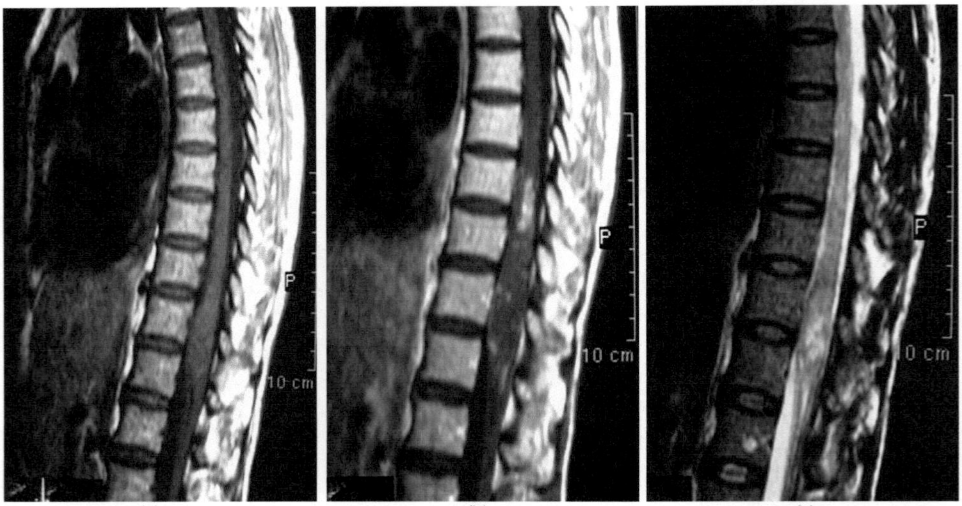

(a) (b) (c)

Figure 3. a-c). Sagital magnetic ressonance imaging in T1 phase (Figure 3a), no contrast T2 phase (Figure 3b), and contrast T2 phase (Figure 3c) in a spinal cord schistosomiasis patient.

8. Imaging examinations

MRIs are very important when investigating spinal cord schistosomiasis and may show important data about the location and extension of the lesions. Although it's not a examination that can define completely the etiology, it may collaborate to differential diagnosis by show-

http://dx.doi.org/10.5772/53771

ing inflammatory lesions and ruling out tumorous lesions. The affected area may present with increased volume or just an increase of paramagnetic contrast caption (Figures 3a, 3b, and 3c). The most frequently found aspect is a granulated pattern that may not be exclusive to, but is highly suggestive of, spinal cord schistosomiasis (Figures 4 and 5). A CT picture has a lower sensibility and, in some cases, may show evidence of increased volume or just high contrast caption [30, 38, 39, 41, 43, 44, 50, 68-71].

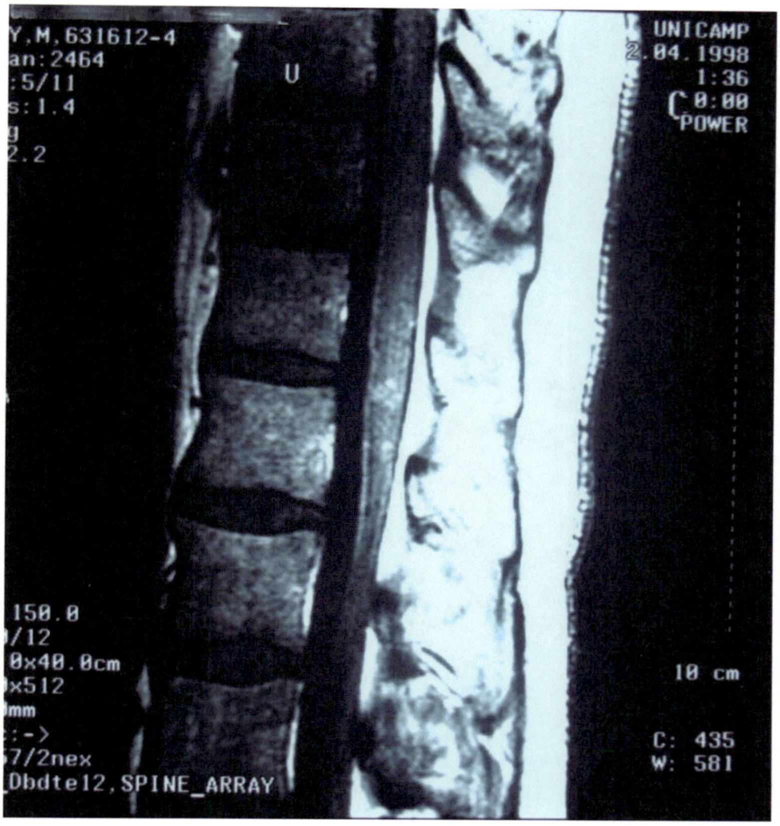

Figure 4. Sagital magnetic ressonance imaging (T2 phase) in a spinal cord schistosomiasis patient. It is observed a granular impregnation of gadolinium magnetic contrast in thoracic-lumbar spinal cord.

9. Laboratory examinations

Nonspecific examinations may suggest the etiology in a clinically suggestive patient. Routine CSF examination may show alterations in a high percentage of the cases, such as increase in proteins in 95% and of leukocytes in 98% of the cases, generally with predominance of lymphocytes and presence of eosinophil granulocytes in 40.8% of the cases

[28]. Despite being highly suggestive of spinal cord schistosomiasis, pelocytoses, high protein concentration and eosinophilia in CSF are not always present [28].

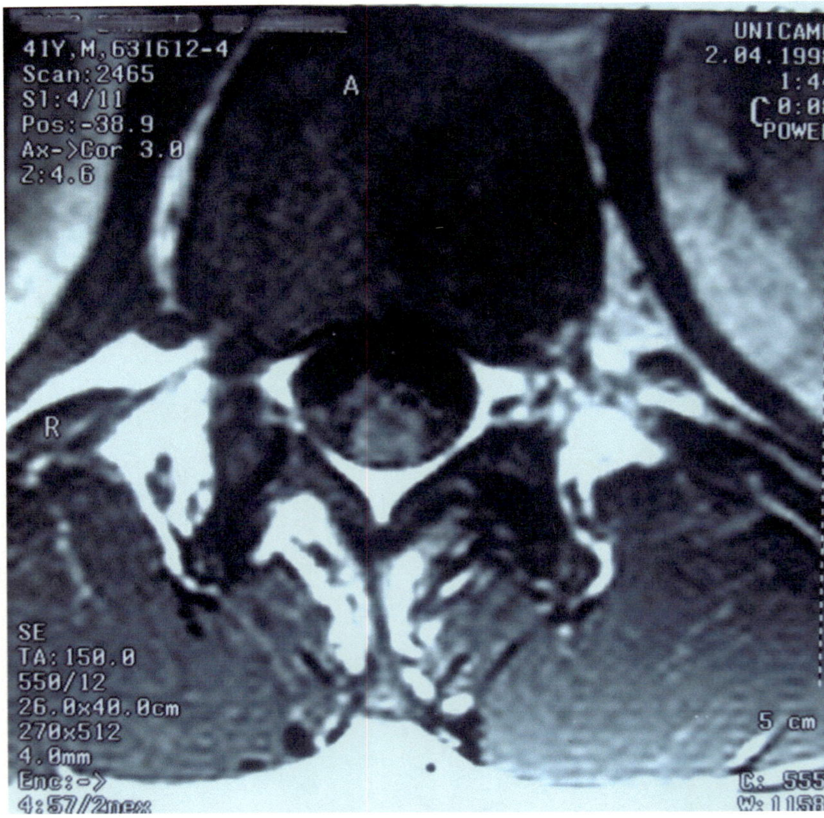

Figure 5. T2 phase axial magnetic ressonance imaging in a spinal cord schistosomiasis patient. It is observed a hypersignal in the thoracic-lumbar spinal cord levels.

Identifying the *Schistosoma* infection through the presence of eggs in the feces (*S. mansoni* and *S. japonicum*) or urine (*S. haematobium*) presents less sensitivity than immunological examinations. In the case of *S. mansoni*, sensitivity varies depending on the methodology and the number of samples being 15.4% [36], 40.0% [26], or 42.5% [42]. Among the several techniques for parasitological examinations, the one which presents the highest sensitivity for *S. mansoni* is Kato-Katz. A study in which 3 to 5 serial fecal samples were collected detected eggs in the feces of 59.4% of the patients [51]. Rectal biopsy, when identifying eggs, shows a positivity ranging from 57.5% [42] to 88,9% [51]. Given that parasitological examinations may be considered to have 100% specificity, any of these tests returning a positive must be considered proof of *Schistosoma* infection, but it may not exclude schistosomiasis when results come back negative.

There are several immunological examination techniques to be used in the serum or CSF. The most used ones try to reveal the presence of antibodies which are specific for soluble egg antigens (SEAs), antigens from the digestive tube of adult worms, or antigens from cercariae. The most used serology techniques are ELISA (Enzyme-linked immunosorbent assay) or indirect immunofluorescence assay. Immunological blood examinations have a sensitivity varying between 80% and 97% and when tested on CSF sensitivity may vary between 56% to 97% (22, 26, 35, 68, 69, 72]. Immunological examinations must be considered as strong evidence of active *Schistosoma* infection, even though many patients who have been cured of the parasites still test positive for a long time and also that there is a chance of cross-reaction with other parasites. Biopsying the medulla is only done, nowadays, in cases when after extensive investigation, the need to rule out tumors is still present [26, 51, 68, 69, 72, 73]. It becomes apparent that no examination may be considered as gold standard for the diagnosis of *Schistosoma* infection and, therefore, analysis of specific examinations must occur alongside analysis of clinical and epidemiological aspects. Also, results from imaging examinations and presence of eosinophil granulocytes in CSF or eosinophilia in peripheral blood must be considered.

A proper investigation must be done to exclude other causes for the medullar and/or radicular lesion, such as bacterial infections (e.g. tuberculosis, syphilis, abscesses), viral infections (e.g. cytomegalovirus, poliovirus, enterovirus, HZV, HSV-1, HSV-2, HIV, HTLV-I) parasitic diseases (e.g. cysticercosis, toxoplasmosis), fungal infections or non-infectious, such as neoplasia, systemic lupus erythematosus, auto-immune vasculitis, diabetic vasculitis, B12 vitamin deficiency, multiple sclerosis, Guillan-Barré Syndrome, among others [26, 51, 68, 69, 72, 73].

10. Treatment

Treatment is done through the use of corticosteroids and schistosomicides. The corticosteroids will diminish the inflammation and lead to regression of the granuloma, being even more important than the schistosomicide. The latter will eliminate the egg production by killing the adult worms and indirectly diminish the production of soluble egg antigens, which are important stimuli for the granulomas. In a few cases, surgical procedures may be necessary to decompress medullar structures. In other cases, treatment is clinical [26, 51, 73]. The schistosomicide may be oxamniquine (15 mg/kg dose for adults and 20 mg/kg for children with up to 5 years of age) or praziquantel (60 mg/kg for children with up to 15 years of age and 50 mg/kg for adults), both in a single dose [73]. The corticosteroid dose is the equivalent to prednisone 1 mg/kg/day, and must be administered for 6 months, with careful suspension, given that patients may present relapses during the process.

In addition, complementary care involves adequate integral approach with psychosocial rehabilitation and motor physical therapy, intermittent bladder checking, prevention of pressure ulcers, among others. Special care must be taken regarding urodynamic aspects [26, 70, 73]. The use of laxatives or enema may be needed for patients with fecal retention.

11. Prognosis

Evolution depends, fundamentally, on early diagnosis and care, better prognosis being associated with an early introduction of the treatment, and particularly the introduction of glucocorticoids [26]. Although symptoms and urological functional alterations do not always respond well to adequate treatment, despite its being started precociously [26, 70, 74, 75]. Patients may recover motor function, sensitivity, sphincter and erectile function control, or they may end up with any combination of absence or recovery of some of the aforementioned functions. Urodynamic alterations have not shown significant improvement in patients who underwent protocol treatment. Ferrari and colleagues (2004) found complete recovery in 31.7% (20) of the patients, 28.3% (18) of the patients presented partial recovery with no functional limitation, 25.4% (16) patients presented partial recovery with functional limitation, and 14.3% (9) of the patients did not improve at all [51]. There were no deaths in this case series. Among the sequelae are paraplegia, paraparesis, dysfunction in the bladder or anal sphincter, sexual dysfunction, definitive sensitivity loss in the affected areas or even paraesthesia and dysesthesia [26, 30, 51]. Detailed studies on the urological aspects, done by Lima (2004) in the Hospital da Restauração in Recife, PE, show that after 9 months of treatment 52 (80%) of 65 patients, showed alterations in urodynamic examinations and 45 (69.2%) showed alterations in voiding cystourethrogram [74].

12. Perspectives

Several factors can actively contribute to the increase in the identification of spinal cord schistosomiasis cases, such as: improvement in diagnostic resources, increase in ecotourism activities with greater exposure of the population to risk of infection, growth of the transmission area, even in urban areas, and lowering of high parasitical loads, without diminishing of the global prevalence of schistosomiasis. There is need of investing in the study of spinal cord schistosomiasis, focusing epidemiological aspects such as: prevalence and incidence, relations between general schistosomiasis incidence and spinal cord schistosomiasis, prevalence and incidence in areas of high and low endemicity, and predisposing factors. Despite how successful controlling the hepatosplenic and cardiopulmonary forms has been throughout the years, control instruments used currently have not shown themselves as sufficient to control the spinal cord schistosomiasis problem. More studies are needed for improving the understanding on the real prevalence of the medullary forms of schistosomiasis. Changes in the Health Surveillance Systems are needed to improve control of schistosomiasis, aiming at a better understanding of the schistosomotic morbidity, particularly that of spinal cord schistosomiasis. It is not surprising that schistosomiasis control politics, based on parasitical diagnostic and treatment of the infected, have not been able to reduce the morbidity of the disease due to medullar lesions, since most patients who present this form of schistosomiasis have low worm burdens and present with negative fecal examinations. To reach effective control of spinal cord schistosomiasis, the introduction of more sensitive diagnostic methods and the development of more effective medicines for diagnosis and

http://dx.doi.org/10.5772/53771

treatment of mild forms of schistosomiasis with low worm burdens will be needed in the basic health systems. For an initial diagnosis, the possibility of immediate introduction of serology as a diagnostic instrument in the Basic Health Units. This examination can be used as diagnostic in those patients who are still untreated. But more studies will be necessary for the development of more effective medicines and of more sensitive methods for parasitological removal. It is also important to disclose the occurrence of this form of schistosomiasis, as well as capacitating professionals for attending these patients, particularly in endemic areas and recently formed focus points. A secondary gain of disclosing information on the existence of severe forms may be the population increase in attendance to control measures for this disease.

Differential diagnosis:
• Bacterial infections: tuberculosis, syphilis, abscesses, Lyme's disease. • Viral infections: cytomegalovirus, poliovirus, enterovirus, HZV, HSV-1, HSV-2, HIV, HTLV, EBV, HBV. • Other infections: cysticercosis, toxoplasmosis, Chagas disease, fungal infections • Non-infectious: neoplasia, systemic lupus erythematosus, auto-immune vasculitis, diabetic vasculitis, B12 deficiency, multiple sclerosis, polyradiculopathy, Guillan-Barré Syndrome, spinal disc herniation, syringomyelia
Typical clinical manifestation:
• Lumbar pain with or without radiation to lower limbs • Paraesthesia or diminishing of lower limb sensitivity • Paraparesis or paraplegia • Anal and bladder sphincter dysfunction • Evolution is generally acute or subacute (between 2 to 60 days)
Presumptive diagnosis:
• Low thoracic or high lumbar medullar symptoms, • Proof of exposure to *Schistosoma ssp* through parasitological or immunological methods and • Exclusion of other causes for myelitis
Typical epidemiological profile of patients with spinal cord schistosomiasis:
• Ages between 15 and 50 • Predominantly male • Low worm burden • Patients thus far do not present symptomatic schistosomiasis or present intestinal and hepatointestinal forms (IS or HIS) • Patients may reside in endemic areas or non-endemic areas, with eventual exposure to risk of infection

Acknowledgements

A special acknowledgment is dedicated to Luana Hughes Freitas for the discussion of the central ideas, inspiration and encouragement for the production of this document. The authors also acknowledge Nicole Montenegro, Marcela Montenegro Coelho e Bruno Montenegro Coelho for their dedication and support for studies in medullary neuroschistosomiasis. Acknowledgment is also due to Professor Luciano de Souza Queiroz, Department of Pathology, FCM-UNICAMP who produced the images of optical microscopy.

Author details

André Ricardo Ribas Freitas[1] and Rodrigo Nogueira Angerami[2]

1 Municipal Secretary of Health of Campinas and Department of Public Health State, Faculty of Medical Sciences, University of Campinas – UNICAMP, Campinas-SP, Brazil

2 Municipal Secretary of Health of Campinas and Department of Clinical Medicine, Faculty of Medical Sciences, State University of Campinas – UNICAMP, Campinas-SP, Brazil

References

[1] World Health Organization DoCoTD. Reports of the WHO informal consultation on schistosomiasis control, WHO/CDS/CPC/SIP/99.2. Geneva, WHO, 1998.

[2] World Health Organization (WHO) http://www.who.int/mediacentre/factsheets/fs115/en/index.html (accessed 7 September 2012)

[3] World Health Organization. The Control of Schistosomiasis. Geneva, 1993.

[4] World Health Organization. Report of informal consultation on schistosomiasis in low transmission areas: control strategies and criteria for elimination. Geneva, 2001.

[5] World Health Organization. Prevention and control of schistosomiasis and soil-transmited helminthiasis. Geneva, 2002.

[6] Thors C, Holmblad P, Maleki M, Carlson J, Linder E. Schistosomiasis in Swedish travellers to sub-Saharan Africa: Can we rely on serology? Scand J Infect Dis 2006; 38(9):794-799.

[7] Agbessi CA, Bourvis N, Fromentin M, Jaspard M, Teboul F, Bougnoux ME, Hanslik T. Acute schistosomiasis in French travellers. Rev Med Interne 2006; 27(8):595-599.

[8] Grandiere-Perez L, Ansart S, Paris L, Faussart A, Jaureguiberry S, Grivois JP, Klement E, Bricaire F, Danis M, Caumes E. Efficacy of praziquantel during the incubation and invasive phase of Schistosoma haematobium schistosomiasis in 18 travelers. Am J Trop Med Hyg 2006; 74(5):814-818.

[9] Ansart S, Perez L, Vergely O, Danis M, Bricaire F, Caumes E: Illnesses in travelers returning from the tropics: a prospective study of 622 patients. J Travel Med 2005; 12(6):312-318.

[10] Greenwald B. Schistosomiasis: implications for world travelers and healthcare providers. Gastroenterol Nurs 2005; 28(3):203-205.

[11] Cantiniaux S, Serratrice J, De Roux-Serratrice C, Disdier P, Perez L, Bricaire F, Caumes E, Mary C, Weiller PJ. A group fever: safari's fever. Rev Med Interne 2004; 25(12):931-933.

[12] Ranque S, Gazin P, Delmont J. Schistosomiasis and tourism in the Dogon country, Mali. Med Trop (Mars) 2004; 64(1):31-32.

[13] Grobusch MP, Muhlberger N, Jelinek T, Bisoffi Z, Corachan M, Harms G, Matteelli A, Fry G, Hatz C, Gjorup I, Schmid ML, Knobloch J, Puente S, Bronner U, Kapaun A, Clerinx J, Nielsen LN, Fleischer K, Beran J, da CS, Schulze M, Myrvang B, Hellgren U. Imported schistosomiasis in Europe: sentinel surveillance data from TropNetEurop. J Travel Med 2003; 10(3):164-169.

[14] Gryseels B, Polman K, Clerinx J, Kestens L. Human schistosomiasis. Lancet 2006; 368(9541):1106-1118.

[15] Lambertucci JR, Sousa-Pereira SR, Silva LC. Myeloradiculopathy in acute schistosomiasis mansoni. Rev Soc Bras Med Trop 2005; 38(3):277-278.

[16] Jesus AR, Silva A, Santana LB, Magalhaes A, de Jesus AA, de Almeida RP, Rego MA, Burattini MN, Pearce EJ, Carvalho EM. Clinical and immunologic evaluation of 31 patients with acute schistosomiasis mansoni. J Infect Dis 2002; 185(1):98-105.

[17] Lambertucci JR, Serufo JC, Gerspacher-Lara R, Rayes AA, Teixeira R, Nobre V, Antunes CM. Schistosoma mansoni: assessment of morbidity before and after control. Acta Trop 2000; 77(1):101-109.

[18] Horak P, Dvorak J, Kolarova L, Trefil L. Trichobilharzia regenti, a pathogen of the avian and mammalian central nervous systems. Parasitology 1999; 119 (Pt 6):577-581.

[19] Kolarova L, Horak P, Cada F. Histopathology of CNS and nasal infections caused by Trichobilharzia regenti in vertebrates. Parasitol Res 2001; 87(8):644-650.

[20] Hradkova K, Horak P. Neurotropic behaviour of Trichobilharzia regenti in ducks and mice. J Helminthol 2002; 76(2):137-141.

[21] Ferrari TC. Spinal cord schistosomiasis. A report of 2 cases and review emphasizing clinical aspects. Medicine (Baltimore) 1999; 78(3):176-190.

[22] Silva LC, Maciel PE, Ribas JG, Pereira SR, Serufo JC, Andrade LM, Antunes CM, Lambertucci JR. Mielorradiculopatia esquistossomótica. Rev Soc Bras Med Trop 2004; 37(3).261-272.

[23] Faust EC. An inquiry into the ectopic lesions in schistosomiasis. Am J Trop Med 1948; 28:175-199.

[24] Kane CA, Most H. Schistosomiasis of the central nervous system: experiences in World War II and review of the literature. Arch Neurol Psychiatry 1948; 59:141-183.

[25] Scrimgeour EM, Gajdusek DC. Involvement of the central nervous system in Schistosoma mansoni and S. haematobium infection. A review. Brain 1985; 108 (Pt 4): 1023-1038.

[26] Freitas ARR, Oliveira ACP, Silva LJ. Schistosomal myeloradiculopathy in a low-prevalence area: 27 cases (14 autochthonous) in Campinas, São Paulo, Brazil. Mem. Inst. Oswaldo Cruz. 2010 July; 105(4): 398-408.

[27] Center of Disease Control. Acute schistosomiasis with transverse myelitis in American students returning from Kenya. MMWR Morb Mortal Wkly Rep 1984; 33(31): 445-447.

[28] Livramento JA, Machado LR, da Silva LC, Spina-Franca A. Cerebrospinal fluid syndrome in neuroschistosomiasis. Arq Neuropsiquiatr 1985; 43(4):372-377.

[29] Haribhai HC, Bhigjee AI, Bill PL, Cosnett JE. Schistosoma in the spinal cord. J Neurol Neurosurg Psychiatry 1988; 51(1):158.

[30] Peregrino AJ, de Oliveira SP, Porto CA, Santos LA, de Menezes EE, Silva AP, Brito AL, Pinheiro SP, Pinheiro S, Dias AB. Meningomielorradiculite por Schistosoma mansoni: protocolo de investigação e registro de 21 casos. Arq Neuropsiquiatr 1988; 46(1):49-60.

[31] Bloom K, Freed MM. Paraplegia from schistosomiasis. Paraplegia 1990; 28(7):455-459.

[32] Chen AW, Alam MH, Williamson JM, Brawn LA. An unusually late presentation of neuroschistosomiasis. J Infect 2006; 53(3):155-158.

[33] Camargos ST, Dantas FR, Teixeira AL. Schistosomal myelopathy mimicking spinal cord neoplasm. Scand J Infect Dis 2005; 37(5):365-367.

[34] Kamel MH, Murphy M, Kelleher M, Aquilina K, Lim C, Marks C. Schistosomiasis of the spinal cord presenting as progressive myelopathy. Case report. J Neurosurg Spine 2005; 3(1):61-63.

[35] Tesser E, Reis ML, Borelli P, Matas SL, Reis Filho JB. Líquido cefalorraquidiano no diagnóstico da esquistossomose raquimedular. Arq Neuropsiquiatr 2005; 63(3A): 661-665.

[36] Carod Artal FJ, Vargas AP, Horan TA, Marinho PB, Coelho Costa PH. Schistosoma mansoni myelopathy: clinical and pathologic findings. Neurology 2004; 63(2): 388-391.

[37] Carod-Artal FJ, Vargas AP. Myelopathy due to Schistosoma mansoni. A description of two cases and review of the literature. Rev Neurol 2004; 39(2):137-141.

[38] Artal FJ, Mesquita HM, Gepp RA, Antunes JS, Kalil RK. Neurological picture. Brain involvement in a Schistosoma mansoni myelopathy patient. J Neurol Neurosurg Psychiatry 2006; 77(4):512.

[39] Freitas ARR, Oliveira ACP, Faria AV. Quatro casos de mielopatia esquistossomótica em áreas de baixa prevalência na região de Campinas-SP. Rev Soc Bras Med Trop 2002; 35 (suppl 1):217.

[40] Grand S, Movet E, Le Bas JF. Case report: spinal cord schistosomiasis, MRI findings. Clin Radiol 1996; 51(10):739-740.

[41] Leite CC, Souza AF, Valente M, Araujo MA, Jinkins JR. Clinics in diagnostic imaging (52). Spinal cord schistosomiasis. Singapore Med J 2000; 41(8):417-419.

[42] Peregrino AJ, Puglia PM, Nobrega JP, Livramento JA, Marques-Dias MJ, Scaff M. Esquistossomose medular: análise de 80 casos. Arq Neuropsiquiatr 2002; 60(3-A): 603-608.

[43] Saleem S, Belal AI, el-Ghandour NM. Spinal cord schistosomiasis: MR imaging appearance with surgical and pathologic correlation. AJNR Am J Neuroradiol 2005; 26(7):1646-1654.

[44] Sanelli PC, Lev MH, Gonzalez RG, Schaefer PW. Unique linear and nodular MR enhancement pattern in schistosomiasis of the central nervous system: report of three patients. AJR Am J Roentgenol 2001; 177(6):1471-1474.

[45] Richter J. The impact of chemotherapy on morbidity due to schistosomiasis. Acta Trop 2003; 86(2-3):161-183.

[46] Scrimgeour EM. Non-traumatic paraplegia in northern Tanzania. Br Med J (Clin Res Ed) 1981; 283(6297):975-978.

[47] Joubert J, Fripp PJ, Hay IT, Davel GH, van Graan ES. Schistosomiasis of the spinal cord--underdiagnosed in South Africa? S Afr Med J 1990; 77(6):297-299.

[48] Scrimgeour EM. Schistosomiasis of the spinal cord--underdiagnosed in South Africa. S Afr Med J 1991; 79(11):680.

[49] Naus CW, Chipwete J, Visser LG, Zijlstra EE, van LL. The contribution made by Schistosoma infection to non-traumatic disorders of the spinal cord in Malawi. Ann Trop Med Parasitol 2003; 97(7):711-721.

[50] Peregrino AJ, Puglia PM, Bacheschi LA, Hirata MT, Brotto MW, Nobrega JP, Scaff M. Diagnosis of schistosomiasis of the spinal cord: contribution of magnetic resonance imaging and electroneuromyography. Arq Neuropsiquiatr 2002; 60(3-A):597-602.

[51] Ferrari TC, Moreira PR, Cunha AS. Spinal cord schistosomiasis: a prospective study of 63 cases emphasizing clinical and therapeutic aspects. J Clin Neurosci 2004; 11(3): 246-253.

[52] Araújo KCGM, Silva CR, Santos AGA, Barbosa CS, Ferrari TCA. Clinical-epidemiologic profile of the schistosomal myeloradiculopathy in Pernambuco, Brazil. Mem. Inst. Oswaldo Cruz [serial on the Internet]. 2010; 105(4): 454-459.

[53] Gonçalves EC, Fonseca AP, Pittella JE. Frequency of schistosomiasis manson,i of its clinicopathological forms and of the ectopic locations of the parasite in autopsies in Belo Horizonte, Brazil. J Trop Med Hyg 1995; 98(5):289-295.

[54] Pittella JE. Neuroschistosomiasis. Brain Pathol 1997; 7(1):649-662.

[55] Pittella JE. The relation between involvement of the central nervous system in schistosomiasis mansoni and the clinical forms of the parasitosis. A review. J Trop Med Hyg 1991; 94(1):15-21.

[56] Vidal, CHF; Gurgel FV; Ferreira MLB, Azevedo-Filho HRC. Epidemiological aspects in neuroschistosomiasis. Arq. Neuro-Psiquiatr. 2010; 68(1): 72-75.

[57] Junker J, Eckardt L, Husstedt I. Cervical intramedullar schistosomiasis as a rare cause of acute tetraparesis. Clin Neurol Neurosurg 2001; 103(1):39-42.

[58] Drumond S C, Silva LCS, Amaral RS, Sousa-Pereira RS, Antunes CM, Lambertucci JR. Morbidity of schistosomiasis mansoni in the state of Minas Gerais, Brazil. Mem Inst Oswaldo cruz 2006; 101(suppl. I):37-40.

[59] Queiroz LS, Nucci A, Facure NO, Facure JJ. Massive spinal cord necrosis in schistosomiasis. Arch Neurol 1979; 36(8):517-519.

[60] Batson OV. The function of the vertebral veins and their role in the spread of metastases. Ann of Surgery 1940; 112(1):138-149.

[61] Pittella JE, Lana-Peixoto MA. Brain involvement in hepatosplenic schistosomiasis mansoni. Brain 1981; 104(3):621-632.

[62] Pittella JE. Partial hypotrophy of the posterior and lateral columns of the spinal cord, representing a sequela of schistosomiasis mansoni: report of an autopsied case and a review of the literature. Clin Neuropathol 1989; 8(6):257-262.

[63] Pearce EJ, Kane M, Sun J, Taylor J, McKee AS, Cervi L. Th2 response polarization during infection with the helminth parasite Schistosoma mansoni. Immunol Rev 2004; 201:117-126.

[64] Stadecker MJ, Asahi H, Finger E, Hernandez HJ, Rutitzky LI, Sun J. The immunobiology of Th1 polarization in high-pathology schistosomiasis. Immunol Rev 2004; 201:168-179.

[65] Wynn TA, Thompson RW, Cheever AW, Mentink-Kane MM. Immunopathogenesis of schistosomiasis. Immunol Rev 2004; 201:156-167.

[66] Ferrari TC, Moreira PR, Sampaio MJ, da Cunha AS, de Oliveira JT, Gazzinelli G, Correa-Oliveira R. Intrathecal cytokines in spinal cord schistosomiasis. J Neuroimmunol 2006; 177(1-2):136-141.

[67] Van LH, Perquin WV. Spinal cord schistosomiasis. J Neurol Neurosurg Psychiatry 2000; 69(5):690-691.

[68] Ferrari TC. Involvement of central nervous system in the schistosomiasis. Mem Inst Oswaldo Cruz 2004; 99(5 Suppl 1):59-62.

[69] Carod Artal, FJ. Cerebral and Spinal Schistosomiasis. Journal Name: Current Neurology and Neuroscience Reports Url: http://dx.doi.org/10.1007/s11910-012-0305-4. (accessed 7 September 2012)

[70] Silva LC, Maciel PE, Ribas JG, Souza-Pereira SR, Antunes CM, Lambertucci JR. Treatment of schistosomal myeloradiculopathy with praziquantel and corticosteroids and evaluation by magnetic resonance imaging: a longitudinal study. Clin Infect Dis 2004; 39(11):1618-1624.

[71] Faria AV, Cerqueira EMFP, Reis F, Pirani C, Damasceno BP, Menezes-Neto JR, Zanardi VA. Apresentações da esquistossomose no sistema nervoso central: correlação clinica e radiológica. Radiol Bras 2002; 35(1):47-50.

[72] Ferrari TC, Moreira PR, Oliveira RC, Ferrari ML, Gazzinelli G, Cunha AS. The value of an enzyme-linked immunosorbent assay for the diagnosis of schistosomiasis mansoni myeloradiculopathy. Trans R Soc Trop Med Hyg 1995; 89(5):496-500.

[73] Brasil. Ministério da Saúde. Guia de vigilância epidemiológica e controle da mielorradiculopatia esquistossomótica. Brasília - DF, 2006.

[74] Lima P. Análise das alterações funcionais vésico-esfincterianas em pacientes com mielopatia esquistossomótica mansônica antes e após o tratamento medicamentoso da doença. PhD thesis. Universidade Federal de São Paulo - UNIFESP, 2004.

[75] Gomes CM, Trigo-Rocha F, Arap MA, Gabriel AJ, aor de FJ, Arap S. Schistosomal myelopathy: urologic manifestations and urodynamic findings. Urology 2002; 59(2): 195-200.

Chapter 7

Study on *Schistosomiasis mansoni* and Comorbidity with Hepatitis B and C Virus Infection

Maria José Conceição and José Rodrigues Coura

Additional information is available at the end of the chapter

http://dx.doi.org/10.5772/55510

1. Introduction

1.1. Comorbidity of *S. mansoni* infection and hepatitis B

In Brazil, despite decreases in the prevalence rates of schistosomiasis and in the frequency of severe forms, the targets for transmission control have not been reached. This should be taken to be a warning sign indicating that schistosomiasis must not be neglected in this country (Conceição & Coura 2012). It is also important to emphasize that co-infections such as the hepatitis B and C viruses play a role.

One of the few studies involving comorbidity with hepatitis B was conducted by Serufo et al. (1998). Two areas with schistosomiasis infection in Minas Gerais were correlated: one endemic and the other, a controlled non-endemic area, where it was shown that schistosomiasis did not change the course of hepatitis B. This had previously been emphasized by Andrade (1965) and Prince (1970), in studies on patients in different geographical regions.

Lyra et al. (1976) compared cases of hepatosplenic schistosomiasis (HSS) and control cases of the hepatointestinal form of the disease, including cases with a variety of illnesses. They found that the patients with HSS were carriers for HBsAg more frequently than the other groups were. Bassily et al. (1979, 1983) detected hepatitis B surface antigen in cases of hepatosplenic schistosomiasis. Pereira et al. (1994) did not find any significant difference in the frequency of these markers for hepatitis B between patients with the hepatointestinal form of schistosomiasis, the hepatosplenic form and controls. Conceição et al. (1998) evaluated the prognosis for individuals infected with *S. mansoni* and carriers of hepatitis B virus, among patients attended at the Teaching Hospital of the Federal University of Rio de Janeiro, Brazil. Non-significant predominance of HBsAg, anti-HBsAg and anti-HBc was detected among patients with the hepatosplenic form of schistosomiasis, who presented greater severity of clinical evolution, with a higher frequency of hematemesis and/or melena. In addition, development of macronodular cirrhosis was observed, with worse prognosis than for patients with the toxemic and hepatointestinal forms. However, Serufo (2000) considered that this kind of association was a fallacy.

Al-Shamiri et al. (2011) determined the disease prevalence and its relationship with hepatitis B and C viruses among 1484 school children aged between 5 and 16 years in five areas endemic for *S. mansoni* and *S. haematobium*. The overall prevalence was 20.76% for *S. mansoni* and 7.41% for *S. haematobium*. There was a correlation between S. *haematobium* and hepatitis B, but no association between *S. mansoni* infection and the hepatitis B and C viruses.

1.2. Association between *S. mansoni* infection and hepatitis C

In Egypt, HCV together with schistosomal parasite infection is the biggest risk factor for chronic liver disease. In most Egyptian patients, HCV genotype 4 is highly prevalent (Halim et al. 1999).

Kamal et al. (2000a) showed that patients with concomitant HCV and schistosomiasis were characterized by more advanced liver disease, higher HCV RNA titers, higher incidence of cirrhosis and hepatocellular carcinoma, and higher incidence of liver-related morbidity and mortality. Kamal et al. (2000b) concluded that patients with chronic hepatitis C and schistosomiasis co-infection responded poorly to interferon therapy and had higher relapse rates than among patients solely infected with chronic HCV.

However, some authors like Gad et al. (2001) and Kamel et al. (2002), in Egypt, mentioned that there appeared to be no epidemiological association between hepatic schistosomiasis and infection by the hepatitis C virus. Also in Egypt, Madwar et al. (1989) evaluated the hepatosplenic forms of the disease and did not show any correlation with serological indicators for hepatitis.

Lambertucci et al. (2005) emphasized that the studies on comorbidity of schistosomiasis and viral hepatitis lacked representative samples of inhabitants and control groups. They concluded that the evolution to chronic hepatitis and hepatic cirrhosis was related to the natural history of hepatitis.

Conceição et al. (2008) presented previous results from a study developed in Itaobim, a rural area of Minas Gerais, Brazil, with the aim of identifying the clinical repercussions of *S. mansoni* infection associated with hepatitis due to the B and C viruses. There was no statistical difference in the viral hepatitis B and C rates among *S. mansoni* infected patients, in comparison with a control group without positive parasitological examinations. From an investigation in the rural area of Jequitinhonha Valley, in Minas Gerais, Conceição et al. (2009) did not find any positive association between serological indicators for hepatitis B or C and severe clinical forms of Manson's schistosomiasis.

The comorbidities that affect the course and response to anti-hepatitis C therapy include schistosomiasis, iron overload, alcohol abuse and excessive smoking. These co-infections negatively affect the course and outcome of liver disease, often reducing the chance of achieving a sustained virological response with PEGylated interferon and ribavirin treatments. Patients with chronic hepatitis C (CHC) infection and concomitant schistosomiasis respond poorly to IFN therapy and have higher relapse rates than among patients with HCV infection only (El-Zayadi 2009). There was no interaction between *S. mansoni* infection or disease and the prevalence or severity of hepatitis C in surveys that were conducted among 2038 Egyptians and 2120 Kenyans (El-Zayad 2009).

2. Research methods

The research methods used for preparing this chapter were based on articles written by our group and by other authors in the literature on the topic of Epidemiology of Schistosomiasis in Brazil, which were published in journals and books in Brazil and worldwide, and in MSc and PhD theses that are available through the internet, in the Oswaldo Cruz Foundation (Fiocruz) libraries, and in the School of Medicine of the Federal University of Rio de Janeiro (UFRJ). Reference was made to protocols and records used in clinical studies and in endemic areas, among the inhabitants, with clinical specifications and socioeconomic conditions. This work also used statistical analysis methods to evaluate whether the results obtained presented significant differences.

3. Conclusions

- Most authors have not found any positive association between serological indicators for hepatitis B or C and the severe clinical forms of schistosomiasis mansoni;
- Comorbidities such as infections due to the hepatitis B and C viruses may worsen the prognosis for the clinical evolution of hepatosplenic schistosomiasis.

Author details

Maria José Conceição[1,2*] and José Rodrigues Coura[1]

*Address all correspondence to: conceição@ioc.fiocruz.br

1 Department of Preventive Medicine and Postgraduate Infectious and Parasitic Diseases Program, Clementino Fraga Filho Hospital, Federal University of Rio de Janeiro (UFRJ), Brazil

2 Laboratory of Parasitic Diseases, Oswaldo Cruz Institute, Fiocruz, Manguinhos, Rio de Janeiro, Brazil

References

[1] Al-shamiri, A. H, Al-taj, M. A, & Ahmed, A. S. (2011). Prevalence and co-infections of schistosomiasis/hepatitis B and C viruses among school children in endemic areas in Taiz, Yemen. *Asian Pacific Journal of Tropical Medicine* , 4(5), 404-8.

[2] Andrade, Z. (1965). Hepatic Schistosomiasis: morphological aspects. In H Popper, F Schaffner (eds), *Progress in Liver Diseases*, Grune & Stratton, New York. , 228-242.

[3] Barbosa FAS (1966). Morbidade da esquistossomose. *Rev Bras Malariol D Trop 8353357*

[4] Bassily, S, Dunn, M. A, Farid, Z, Kilpatrick, M. E, Masry, A. G, Kamel, I. A, Alamy, M. E, & Murphy, B. L. (1983). Chronic hepatitis B in patients with schistosomiasis mansoni. *J Trop Med Hyg 866771*

[5] Bassily, S, Farid, Z, Highashi, G. L, Kamel, I. A, & Watten, E. L-M. a. s. r. y A. G. RH (1979). Chronic hepatitis B antigenemia in patients with hepatosplenic schistosomiasis. *J Trop Med Hyg 82248251*

[6] Blanton, R. E, Salam, E. A, Kariuki, H. C, Magak, P, Silva, L. K, Muchiri, E. M, Thiongo, F, Abdel-meghid, I. E, Butterworth, A. E, Reis, M. G, & Ouma, J. H. (2002). Population-based differences in Schistosoma mansoni- and hepatitis C-induced disease. *J Infect Dis.* , 185(11), 1644-9.

[7] Chieffi, P. P. (1992). Interrelationship between Schistosomiasis and concomitant diseases. *Mem Inst Oswaldo Cruz 87291296*

[8] Conceição, M. J, & Argento, C. A. Chagas VLA, Takiya CM, Moura DC, Silva SCF. *S. mansoni* Patients Infected with Hepatitis B. (1998). *Mem Inst Oswaldo Cruz*, 93(Suppl. I): , 255-258.

[9] Conceição, M. J, & Coura, J. R. (2012). Epidemiology of Schistosomiasis in Brazil. In: IN: Rokni MB. Schistosomiasis. 1ª. ed. Ed. In Tech. Cap. 9. Available at www.interchopen.com, 183-192.

[10] Conceição, M. J. Oliveira MLA, Silva MLP, Silva IM, Borges-Pereira J. (2005). Correlation of Viral Hepatitits A, B, C, D in Patients Infected with *Schistosoma mansoni* in a rural area from Capitão Andrade, Rio Doce Valley, Minas Gerais, Brazil. Abstracts X International Symposium on Schistosomiasis, Belo Horizonte, Minas Gerais, Brazil. 25-28 September , 134.

[11] Conceição, M. J, & Silva, I. M. Yoshida CFT, Carlôto AE, Melo EV, Lemos EA, Miguel JC, Euzébio JEG, Pires L. (2008). Prevalence of Serological Assays for Viral Hepatitis B and C in Inhabitants from Itaobim, an Endemic Area of Schistosomiasis mansoniin Jequitinhonha Valley, Minas Gerais, Brazil. Abstracts XI International Symposium on Schistosomiasis, Salvador-Bahia, Brazil. 20-22 August , 161.

[12] Coutinho, A. (1979). Fatores relacionados com o desenvolvimento das formas clínicas da esquistossomose mansônica. *Rev Assoc Med Bras 25185188*

[13] Coutinho, A. Domingues ALC (1988). Esquistossomose mansoni. In R Danni, LP Castro (eds), *Gastroenterologia Clínica,* 2nd ed., Ed. Guanabara Koogan, Rio de Janeiro, , 1362-1386.

[14] El-Zayadi, A. (2009). Hepatitis C comorbidities affecting the course and response to therapy. *World J. Gastroenterol.* , 15, 4993-4999.

[15] Gad, A, Tanaka, E, Orii, K, Rokuhara, A, Nooman, Z, Serwah, A. H, Shoair, M, Yoshizawa, K, & Kiyosawa, K. (2001). Relationship between hepatitis C virus infection and Schistosomal liver disease: not simply an additive effect. *J Gastroenterol.* , 36(11), 753-8.

[16] Ghaffar, Y. A, Fattah, S. A, Kamel, M, Badr, R. M, Mahomed, F. F, & Strickland, G. T. (1991). The impact of endemic schistosomiasis on acute viral hepatitis. *Am J Trop Med Hyg 45743750*

[17] Garry, A. B, Dash, R. F, & Gerber, S. MA. (1999). Effect of schistosomiasis and hepatitis on liver disease. *Am J Trop Med Hyg* , 60(6), 915-920.

[18] Hammad, H. A. El-Fattah MMZ, Morris M, Madiner EH, El-Abbasy AA, Soliman AMT(1990). Study on some hepatic functions and prevalence of hepatitis B surface antigenemia in Egyptian children with schistosomiasis hepatic fibrosis. *J Trop Pediat 36126130*

[19] Hyams KC Alamy MEPazzaglia G, El-Ghorab NM, Sidom O, Habib M, Dunn MA (1987). Risk of hepatitis B infection among Egyptians with *Schistosoma mansoni. Am J Trop Med Hyg 3510351039*

[20] Kamal, S. M, Madwar, M. A, Bianchin, L, Tawil, A. F, Fawxy, R, Peters, T, & Rasenack, J. W. (2000a). Clinical virological and histopathological features: long-term follow-up in patients with chronic hepatitis C co-infected with *Schistosoma mansoni. Liver* , 4, 281-289.

[21] Kamal, S. M, Madwar, M. A, Peters, T, Fawzy, R, & Rasenack, J. (2000b). Interferon therapy in patients with hepatitis C and schistosomiasis. *Journal of Hepatology.* , 32, 172-174.

[22] Kamel, K. C, Alamy, M. E, Miller, F. D, Masry, A. G, Zakaris, S, Khattab, M, & Essmat, G. (1994). The epidemiology of *Schistosoma mansoni,* hepatitis B and hepatitis C infection in Egypt. *Ann Trop Med Parasitol 88501509*

[23] Kato, K. (1960). A correct application of the thick-smear technique with cellophane paper cover. A pamphlet, In Komyia Y & Kobayashi A. (eds). Evaluation of Kato thick-smear technique with a cellophane cover for helminth eggs in Feces. *Jap J Med Sci Biol 19*: 58-64., 9.

[24] Katz, N, Chaves, A, & Pellegrino, J. (1972). A simple device for quantitative stool thick-smear technique in schistosomiasis mansoni. *Rev Inst Med Trop São Paulo 4397400*

[25] Lambertucci, J. R. Silva LCS, Voieta I. (2005). Esquistossomose Mansônica. In Coura JR. Dinâmica das Doenças Infecciosas e Parasitárias. 1ª edição. Editora Guanabara Koogan, , 932-946.

[26] Larouze, B, Dazza, M. C, Gaudebout, C, Habib, M, Elamy, M, & Cline, B. (1987). Absence of relationship between *Schistosoma mansoni* and hepatitis B virus infection in the Qalyub Governate- Egypt. *Ann Trop Med Parasitol 81373375*

[27] Lutz, A. e a Schistosomatose segundo observações feitas no Brasil. *Mem Inst Oswaldo Cruz 11121155*

[28] Lyra, L. D, Rebouças, G, & Andrade, Z. (1976). Hepatitis B surface antigen carrier state in hepatosplenic schistosomiasis. *Gastroenterology 71641647*

[29] Madwar, M. A, Tahawy, M, & Strickland, G. T. (1989). There was not relationship between uncomplicated schistosomiasis and hepatitis B infection. *Trans R Soc Trop Med Hyg 83233236*

[30] Pereira LMMBMelo MCV, Lacerda C, Spinelli V, Domingues ALC, Massarolo P, Mies S, Saleh MG, Mcfarlane IG, William R (1994). Hepatitis B virus infection in Schistosomiasis mansoni. *J Med Virol 42203206*

[31] Pessoa, S. B, & Barros, P. S. (1953). Notas sobre a Epidemiologia da esquistossomose mansônica no Estado de Sergipe. *Rev Med Cir São Paulo 13147154*

[32] Prince, A. M. (1970). Prevalence of serum hepatitis related antigen (SH) in different geographic regions. *Am J Trop Med Hyg 19*: 872.

[33] Serufo, J. C. (2000). Association of Hepatitis B and Schistosomiasis: an ecological fallacy. Rev. Soc. Bras. Med. Trop. Abstract-PhD Thesis, Universidade Federal de Minas Gerais-UFMG., 33(1), 103-104.

[34] Serufo, J. C. Antunes CMF, Pinto-Silva RA, Gerspacher-Lara R, Rayes AAM, Drummond SC, Reis CMF, Martins MJ, Mingoti SA, Lambertucci JR. (1998). Chronic Carriers of Hepatitis B Surface Antigen in an Endemic Area for Schistosomiasis mansoni in Brazil. Mem. Inst.Oswaldo Cruz *9* (Suppl. I): , 249-253.

Section 3

Drugs and Vaccines

Chapter 8

Tegument of *Schistosoma mansoni* as a Therapeutic Target

Claudineide Nascimento Fernandes de Oliveira,
Rosimeire Nunes de Oliveira, Tarsila Ferraz Frezza,
Vera Lúcia Garcia Rehder and
Silmara Marques Allegretti

Additional information is available at the end of the chapter

http://dx.doi.org/10.5772/53653

1. Introduction

Schistosomiasis is a parasitic disease with great social impact, being regarded as a relevant public health issue in 76 countries in Africa, Asia, and South and Central Americas [1, 2]. It is one of the main water-borne parasitic diseases in the world and it continues to be a major cause of morbidity and mortality, disabling and killing thousands of people every year. Considering that, both public health bodies and pharmaceutical companies need to more diligent regarding that issue [3, 4].

The parasite that causes schistosomiasis mansoni is the *Schistosoma mansoni,* an intravascular digenetic trematode from the family Schistosomatidae. In Brazil, where only that particular schistosome can be found, there are 25 million people living in endemic areas, from which 4 to 6 million are infected, which makes the country the most affected by intestinal schistosomiasis in all Americas. Popularly known as barriga-d'água (water belly) in Brazil, the disease is transmitted by planorbides from genus *Biomphalaria* [5, 6].

The transmission occurs when an infected definitive host eliminates viable eggs of the parasite through stool, getting in contact with bodies of fresh water and contaminating them. Therefore, the disease is directly related to fast urban growth and lack of resources such as safe water supply and adequate sewage system in peri-urban areas [7]. The pathology of the disease is characterized by having two phases, acute and chronic, which are dependent on the life stage of the parasite, as shown in Figure 1.

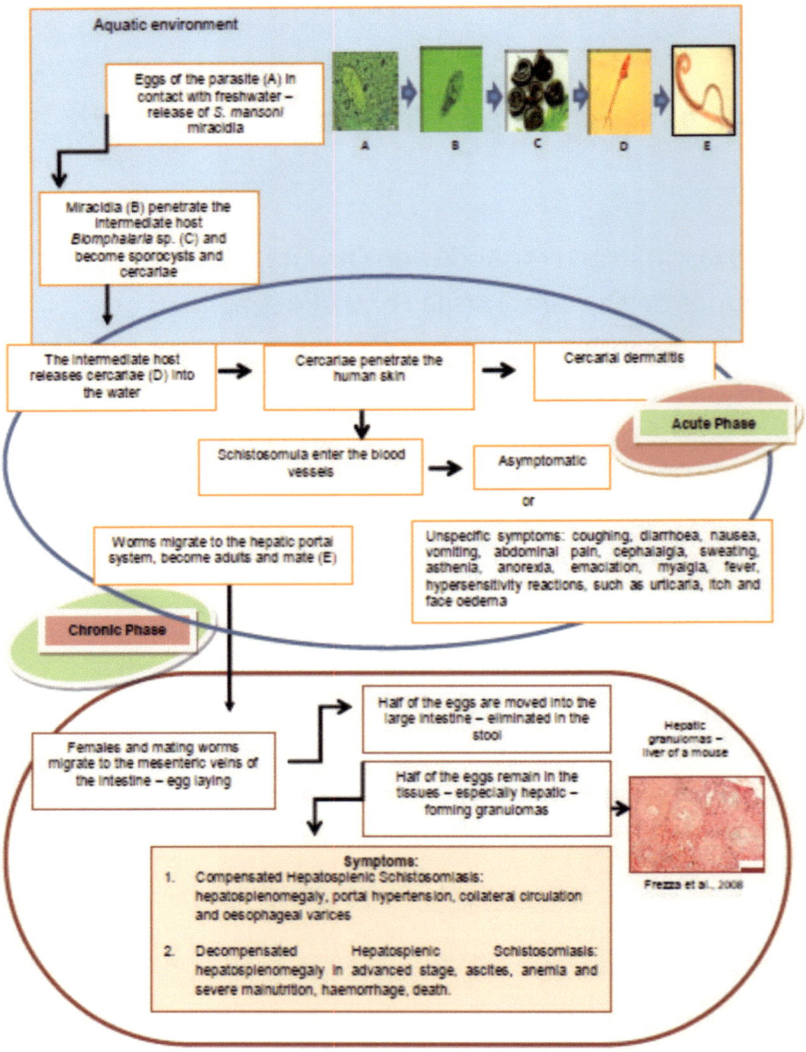

Figure 1. Cycle and pathology of schistosomiasis mansoni.

According to [8], environmental degradation is a determining factor to the dissemination of the disease, even more than poverty and underdevelopment. The authors also consider that some factors contribute to both development and maintenance of schistosomiasis mansoni breeding sites, such as subsistence cultivation; perennial cultivation; flooded areas; meanders and natural channels; springs and taps; environments likely to be polluted by human waste; fish-breeding ponds; ponds or watercourses used for sport fishing, washing of utensils, and bathing; sand deposits on river banks with no vegetation; large debris and garbage deposits and activities along watercourse banks. As a result, the authors believe that the distribution of the disease is not as random as it seems, and that the localities with concentration of cases are associated with human activities that interfere with both landscape structure and human behavior, so there is a relationship between land occupation and health decline. In reference [9], the authors have recently confirmed this hypothesis by reporting the rise of the disease in the state of Bahia (Brazil), particularly in the town of Lauro de Freitas, which full ongoing economic growth is attracting intense human migration, which results in disordered urban occupation and environmental disturbances, increasing the risk of expanding the endemic area. Because of that, schistosomiasis mansoni is considered one of the most critical health issues in Brazil, occurring in 19 states (out of 26 states and one Capitol) [9, 10].

2. Therapeutics of schistosomiasis mansoni: Searching for new alternatives

Several intervention measures can be taken to reduce the morbidity of the disease, as well as, to prevent or interrupt the transmission of the parasite from the mollusk intermediate host to humans. Such measures include chemotherapy, environmental sanitation, mollusk control, safe water supplies, and environmental education.

Chemotherapy provides a double benefit: it reduces both the morbidity caused by the presence of adult worms in the human host and the number of eggs eliminated to the environment [11].

There are only two drugs available for the treatment of schistosomiasis mansoni, i.e., oxamniquine and praziquantel. However, since the former has side effects on the human organism (mutagenic and carcinogenic effects, as well as effects on the central nervous system), its production and commercialization are controlled and reduced. Therefore, praziquantel has been practically the only drug available for that treatment since the 1970s [12-14]. To exacerbate the situation, cases of tolerance and resistance of *S. mansoni* to the treatment with both drugs have been recently reported, which raises the need to develop new drugs and forms of controlling the disease [15-17].

In this context, research with medicinal plants becomes a viable alternative, especially in countries with large biodiversity and rich cultural and ethnic diversity, like Brazil, because of the resulting accumulation of local traditional knowledge, which is passed from generation to generation and includes the use and management of medicinal plants as home remedies [18]. Furthermore, there are about 100,000 catalogued plant species in Brazil, and their active ingredients are mostly unknown, as only 8% of those species were studied regarding their chemical composition and therapeutic properties [19]. In recent years, the scientific community has been conducting *in vitro* and *in vivo* tests to examine a variety of essential oils, extracts and isolated compounds from different species with respect to their schistosomicidal potential.

In the last few years, our research group carried out *in vitro* and *in vivo* tests using three species of Brazilian medicinal plants – *Baccharis trimera* (Less) DC., *Cordia verbenacea* DC and *Phyllanthus amarus* – on adult *S. mansoni* worms. The three species are widely used in Brazilian folk medicine in the forms of infusion and tea on account of their anti-inflammatory properties.

Amongst the several criteria analyzed by our research group to evaluate the therapeutic efficiency of the tested plants, the morphological changes in the tegument of the worms (both males and females) were considered essential, due to the fact that literature reports the damage caused to that structure as cardinal in causing the parasite's death, and studies for the development of new schistosomicidal drugs have been setting it as a target [20].

3. The importance of the tegument of *Schistosoma mansoni*

The tegument of *S. mansoni* plays a key role in its protection against the action of the host's immune system, as it is renovated every six hours [20]. In addition to that, it is capable of absorbing nutrients and molecules and synthesizing some proteins [21-24]. That structure is also extremely important for the success of the infection and the survival of the worm in the host [25-27]. For all those reasons, it has been vastly studied since the end of the 1960s.

3.1. The analysis evolution of the tegument of *S. mansoni*: From optical to electron microscopy

Before microscopy techniques were available for the evaluation of the worm ultrastructure, little was known about the importance of the tegument of *S. mansoni*. The first detailed studies on that structure were carried out in the 1940s, when Gönnert [28], using light microscopy, described the differences between *S. mansoni* males and females, including the fact that males have more and larger thorns.

With the emergence of transmission electron microscopy (TEM) and scanning electron microscopy (SEM) there was a revolution regarding the 'appearance' of the worm and the description of its sexual dimorphism. By using electron beams that either pass through (in the case of TEM) or scan the specimen under analysis (in the case of SEM), electron microscopy, which was developed in the 1930s, had a significantly higher resolving power than optical microscopy, allowing for a detailed observation of samples.

According to [29, 30], *S. mansoni* was the first digenetic trematode to be examined under electron microscopy. For that reason, the ultrastructure of that helminth has been more often studied than the ultrastructure of any other digenetic trematode. By the end of the 1960s and beginning of the 1970s, electron microscopy was used in studies on schistosomiasis mansoni to confirm details of the parasite's tegument and thus allowed for interpretation of the functions of that structure.

In 1968, Hockley [31] described the surface of the worm using SEM, pointing out, for instance, the presence of thorns in the more internal portion of the oral sucker in both sexes, and the fact that the ventral sucker (acetabulum) is longer and more conspicuous in males. Still according to that author, the genital pore was detected in both sexes in the form of an opening placed posteriorly to the ventral sucker. The author also reported the presence of tubercles on the dorsal surface of male worms starting from the posterior portion of the ventral sucker, both sides being covered by thorns. The number of such tubercles starts to decrease from the posterior lateral edges of the dorsal surface.

Furthermore, Hockley [31] observed that in the areas between the tubercles the parasite's surface is rugged, with several grooves, as well as a few isolated thorns. On the male worm lateral edge, which bends to form the gynaecophoric canal, the author noticed the presence of large thorns whose function is to capture the female in the canal. Finally, he noticed that females also presents more thorns at the final portion of their surface, but in less quantity than males. Senft and Gibler [32] termed such thorns sensory papillae.

Using TEM, Hockley and McLaren [33] concluded that the surface of *S. mansoni* consists of two opposite lipid bilayers very close to each other and having the form of a cell membrane. Since the tegument does not have lateral membranes, its cytoplasm extends as a continuous unity, or syncytium, around the body of the worm. According to the authors, that syncytial complex is the main route of nutrient absorption (glucose, amino acids, among others), metabolite excretion (lactic acid and others) and protection against attacks by the host's immune system, whereupon it is a crucial target of drugs with schistosomicidal activity.

From the 1980s on, after the establishment of the therapeutics of schistosomiasis mansoni, TEM and especially SEM were also used in an attempt to clarify the action mechanisms of the drugs used in the treatment for the disease, i.e., oxamniquine and praziquantel.

Becker et al. [34], by means of SEM and TEM, realized that worms subjected to oxamniquine showed tegumental vacuolization. Using SEM, Kohn et al. [35] noticed that the drug was producing changes in the structure of the worm on tegumental, muscular and parenchymal levels, causing bubble-like lesions. Magalhães-Filho et al. [36] also noticed vacuolization, destruction of tubercles in male worms, and surface erosion. Recently, praziquantel has been subjected to further studies because it still is the most used drug in the treatment of all types of schistosomiasis.

Using SEM and TEM, Shaw and Erasmus [37] observed extensive damage to the structure of *S. mansoni* specimens subjected to praziquantel, including vacuolization of the tegument and subtegument of females, and destruction of the tegument and musculature. In males, in addition to vacuolization and destruction of the parenchymal tissue, mainly in the dorsal region, loss of cytoplasm, and structural damages to the musculature could be observed. It was noticed that male worms showed more damage in the tegument than females.

Actually, the action mechanism of praziquantel on *S. mansoni* has yet to be fully understood. On the other hand, there is no doubt that studies using SEM and TEM were important in the search to solve that puzzle.

The morphological changes that praziquantel causes to the tegument and in the sarcoplasmic membranes of the parasite are thought to be followed by an increase of antigen exposure on its surface. The antigens are identified and connected with the host's immune response required to complement the activity of the drug [38, 39]. Therefore, praziquantel is believed to interact with the host's immune system to kill the parasite. The last effect of the drug is the rupture of the surface of the worm, leading to its death [40].

In view of the fact that certain strains of the parasite have proved to be tolerant and resistant to the treatment with oxamniquine and praziquantel, it has become necessary to test new drugs. Electron microscopy has been used since the 1990s to know if such drugs are active against the worm by observing the damages caused to its tegument. Many studies using SEM have shown that drugs active against *S. mansoni* are responsible for severe damage to its tegument.

Some drugs, which had their schistosomicidal activity studied, have proved capable of producing tegumental changes. Albuquerque et al. [41] noticed that imidazole derivatives causes damage to the oral sucker in males, in addition to reducing and disorganizing the tubercles. In females the authors noticed erosion and peeling of the tegument, rupture of the surface membrane, and the complete disappearing of sensory structures.

Manneck et al. [42] observed that mefloquine causes higher degree of changes to the tegument of schistosomula and adult females, including peeling and bubble formation. Tests with that drug have also been carried out with other *Schistosoma* sp. (e.g., *S. japonicum*, which causes intestinal schistosomiasis), and these were the effects described: peeling in males and females, fusion of thorns in males, collapse of the sensory papillae, and erosion on the suckers [43].

In assays carried out with arachidonic acid, El Ridi et al. [44] showed extensive changes in the aspect of tubercles in males, including reduction in size and loss of thorns. The suckers also underwent changes such as oedemas and loss of thorns.

Other authors used SEM to attest the activity of natural compounds on the tegument of the worm. Shuhua et al. [24] reported that artemether, a derivative compound of artemisinin, which is extracted from *Artemisia annua,* causes damage to the tegument of both males and females, including peeling, which was more intense in females – not surprisingly, as artemisinin itself is most effective against females [45]. Oliveira et al. [46] noticed extensive peeling on the tegument of male and female worms, destruction of tubercles, thorns and sensory papillae, and changes in the suckers (oral and ventral) after *in vitro* exposure to essential oil of *Baccharis trimera* over an incubation period of 24 hours.

3.2. *S. mansoni* tegument analysis method

Nowadays, other techniques are being used in an attempt to evaluate the activity of candidate drugs on the tegument of the worm. One of them is confocal laser scanning microscopy (CLSM), which, like SEM, provides three-dimensional images. The confocal microscope was developed in 1950, but it only became popular for analysis of biological samples in the 1970s [47-50].

Moraes et al. [27-51] used confocal laser scanning microscopy to analyze the activity of piplartine (isolated from *Piper tuberculatum*) on the tegument of *S. mansoni* adults and schistosomula, and reported reduction in the quantity of tubercles in males and damage to the surface membrane of schistosomula. Moraes [51] proposed the use of both CLSM and SEM to perform a quantitative analysis (by counting the tubercles in a specific area) of the damage caused to the tegument of worms used in drug testing.

Another way to evaluate tegument damage caused by candidate drugs is to use an inverted optical microscope during *in vitro* assays. Magalhães et al. [52] and Moraes et al. [51], for example, reported damage to the tegument of *S. mansoni* specimens subjected to *in vitro* assays with *Dryopteris* sp. and *Piper tuberculatum*, respectively, considering them either moderate or severe.

Therefore, there are other methods besides electron microscopy to evaluate the activity of a drug or candidate drug on the tegument of *S. mansoni*. Such methods can be classified as qualitative (i.e., it is only possible to notice changes, not to measure them), quantitative (changes can be quantified, i.e., it is possible to count and compare, for instance, the number of tubercles in male worms subjected to the tested sample with the number found in the control group), and qualitative-quantitative (in this case, changes can be both visualized and quantified). Table 1 presents that classification.

Method	Classification	Advantages	Disadvantages	References
Inverted Optical Microscope (used during *in vitro* tests)	Qualitative	- No special preparation is required to visualize the sample -Damages to the tegument can be visualized live, whilst the *in vitro* experiment is carried out -It is possible to analyze a higher range in less time	-Analysis criteria are subjective: damages must be evaluated subjectively, e.g., they are reported as intense, intermediate, moderate, or even absent	[51, 52,53-57]
Confocal Laser Scanning Fluorescence Microscopy	Quantitative	- Allows damages to be quantified through three-dimensional images, especially on the tegument of male worms, where the number of changed or damaged tubercles is counted -Provides images of great contrast even with weakly fluorescent specimens -Three-dimensional images with a resolving power of 0.1-0.2 μm, providing many details of the surface of the worm	-Sample has to be prepared - Expensive - Complex to operate -High-intensity laser light - Chemical labeling	[51]
Transmission Electron Microscopy	Qualitative	- Allows for the analysis not only of damages caused to the tegument of the worm but also of changes in its musculature and internal organs - Excellent resolution (< 0,2 nm)	- Sample preparation is a delicate and difficult work - Tegumental damages cannot be statistically quantified - Expensive	[43, 58, 59]
Scanning Electron Microscopy	Qualitative/ Quantitative	- Three-dimensional images with high angular resolution (~10 nm), providing many details of the surface of the worm - Like in confocal laser scanning fluorescence microscopy, damages to the tegument can be quantified - High-quality three-dimensional images, ideal to analyse the texture, topography and surface of the worm	- Sample has to be prepared - Expensive	[24, 46,58]

Table 1. Methods to analyze damage to the tegument of *S. mansoni* specimens subjected to either *in vitro* or *in vivo* tests *for* evaluation of candidate drugs*:* classification. Sources: [60-63].

Our research group has evaluated the activity of different fractions of *B. trimera, C. verbenacea* and *P. amarus* on the tegument of adult *S. mansoni* males and females using SEM. We understand that this method provides important data regarding tegumentary changes because its high angular resolution provides high-quality images that allow us to analyse the parasite's surface in detail.

4. Methodologies used in scanning electron microscopy for studies of *S. mansoni*

On account of their naturally hydrated condition, biological samples are relatively complex to process, and only hard objects (e.g., seeds) can be observed through SEM with minimum preliminary treatment. Therefore, the preparation of a biological sample for SEM includes various stages [60, 64].

From the first observations using SEM to the present ones, it can be noticed that the methodology for *S. mansoni* worms preparation has significantly varied from one author to the other. Nevertheless, the steps for preparing the worms have always been respected: fixation, washing to remove the excess of fixatives, post-fixation in osmium tetroxide, dehydration at growing concentrations of ethanol, critical point drying, mounting on aluminum stubs, gold sputtering, and observation under a scanning electron microscope. Table 2 shows differences in the methodologies for preparing *S. mansoni* specimens for SEM analysis.

Although some methodologies for preparation of *S. mansoni* samples for SEM use phosphate buffer, some authors use sodium cacodylate buffer. Considering that, an experiment was carried out in order to evaluate possible differences between the use of such biological buffers. A protocol was used, and only the biological buffer was changed:

1. Fixation in Karnovsky (2.5% glutaraldehyde and 4% paraformaldehyde) with buffering pH between 7.0 and 7.3 (adjusted with 0.2 M HCL) with 0.1 M sodium cacodylate buffer solution or 0.1 M phosphate during 48 hours; 2. Washing in 0.1 M sodium cacodylate buffer or 0.1 M phosphate for one hour, changing the solution every 15 minutes; 3. Post-fixation in 1% osmium tetroxide for one hour; 4. Washing in 0.1 M sodium cacodylate buffer or 0.1 M phosphate for 30 minutes, changing the solution every 10 minutes; 5. Dehydration at growing concentrations of ethanol (50% and 70% during 30 minutes, changing the solution after 15 minutes; 90% and 100% during 30 minutes, changing the solution every 10 minutes); 6. Drying of worms in a critical point dryer; 7. Mounting of the samples on aluminum stubs; 8. Gold Sputtering; 9. Observation under a scanning electron microscope

Figures 2 to 7 present images obtained with different buffers. It could be noticed that the samples subjected to phosphate buffer showed inferior fixation as compared to sodium cacodylate, since the worms became malleable and, especially males, seemed to dehydrate. For that reason, sodium cacodylate buffer was used in the subsequent assays. However, it could also be noticed that the use of Karnovsky solution in fixation, as well as the long period in which the samples stayed therein, rendered the worms stiff, friable and hard to manipulate.

The use of 2.5% glutaraldehyde as fixative for a shorter incubation period (24 hours) was, thus, adopted by our group.

Figure 8 shows the standardized protocol that was applied to all SEM assays with the studied plant species, i.e., *B. trimera, C. verbenacea* and *P. amarus.* The samples were mounted on aluminum stubs, placed in a Balzers critical point dryer, model CPD 030, and a Bal-Tec/Balzers sputtering system (Sputter Coater), model SCD 50, and then were analyzed under a Jeol scanning electron microscope, model JSM 5800LV.

Methodology	Type	Advantages	Disadvantages	References
Pre-fixatives	Glutaraldehyde (AG)	- In addition to not causing protein coagulation, AG is incorporated into tissues (additive fixative), promoting good structural fixation - Maintains good fixation quality up to 30 days if kept at -20°C	- When kept in alkaline medium at 4°C, there can be polymerisation, which reduces the osmolarity of the solution	[65-67]
	Formalin	- Low cost	- Methanol concentration varies from 11% to 16%, extracting most of cytosol and cell membrane, providing bad fixation conditions	[68,69]
	Karnovsky (2.5% glutaraldehyde and 4% paraformaldehyde)	- Paraformaldehyde penetrates 5 times faster than AG, but, because its fixation power is lower, it promotes a weaker initial stabilization, which will then be complemented by AG. As a result, the solution will have more osmolarity	- Combined use of two toxic substances	[70-72]
Buffer solution	Sodium cacodylate	- Absence of phosphate ions that can interfere with cytochemical studies - Preservation of the activity of certain enzymes and resistance to contamination, as it contains arsenic	- Highly toxic, partially for having arsenic in its composition - Its disposal demands special care	[65, 67, 70,71]
	Phosphate	- It is more physiological than sodium cacodylate buffer, not having toxicity	- Can produce artefacts in the form of electron-dense particles	[24,41]

Table 2. Methodological differences for the preparation of *S. mansoni* specimens for SEM. Sources: [73, 74].

Sodium Cacodylate Group – mated worms

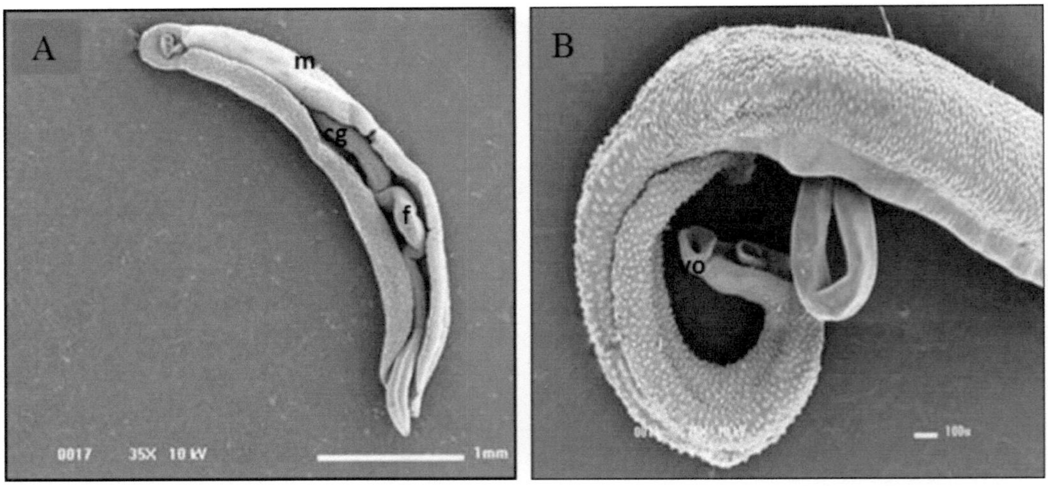

Figure 2. Scanning electron microscopy of adult *S. mansoni* using sodium cacodylate buffer. A-B – mated *S. mansoni* worms; m: male worm; f: female worm; cg: gynaecophoric canal, vo: oral sucker, Va: ventral sucker.

Sodium Cacodylate Group – Tegument

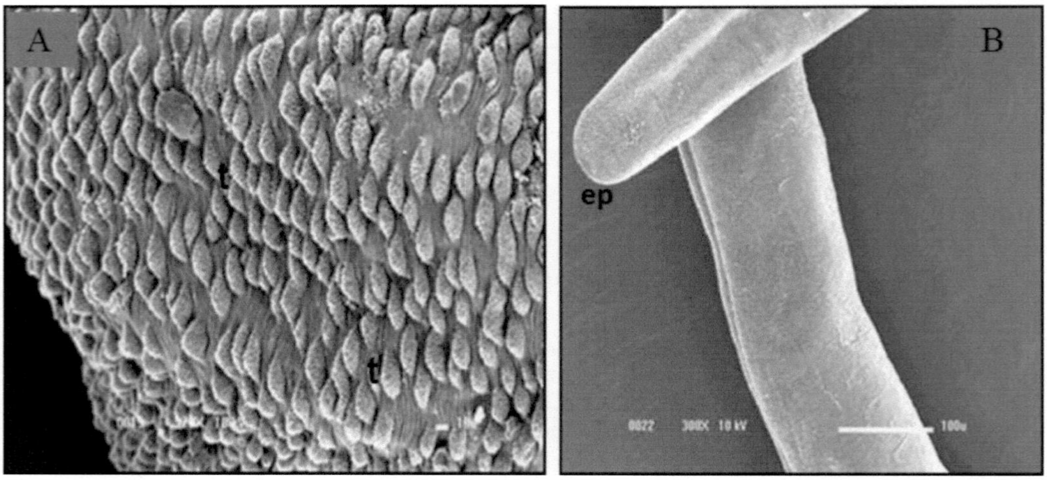

Figure 3. Scanning electron microscopy of the tegument of adult *S. mansoni* worms using sodium cacodylate buffer. **A** – tegument of male worm; **B** – tegument of female worm. **t**. tubercles. **ep** – excretory pore.

Sodium Cacodylate Group – Suckers

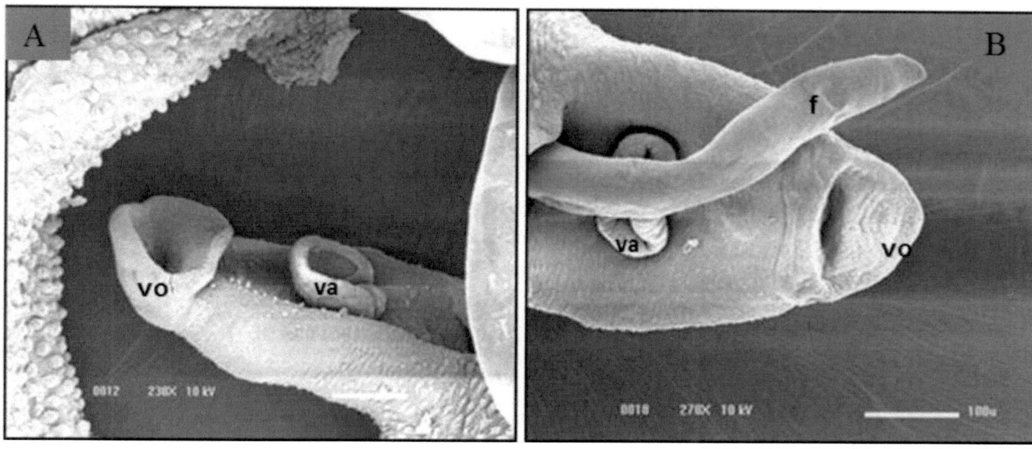

Figure 4. Scanning electron microscopy of *S. mansoni* male worm suckers using sodium cacodylate buffer. vo. oral sucker; va. ventral sucker; f. female worm.

Phosphate Group – Mated Worms

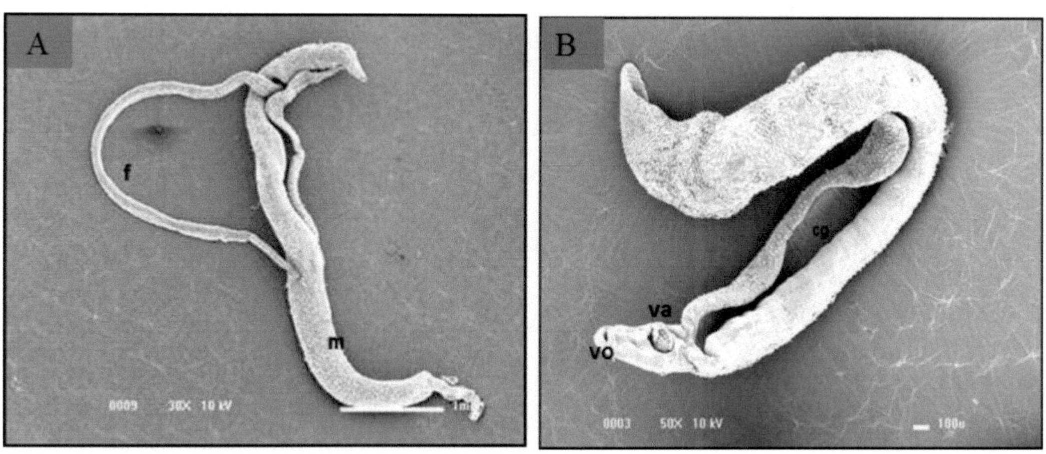

Figure 5. SEM of adult *S. mansoni* worms using sodium phosphate buffer. A- male worm; **f-** female worm; B- male worm; **vo-** oral sucker; **va**- ventral sucker. **cg**- gynaecophoric canal.

Phosphate Group – Tegument

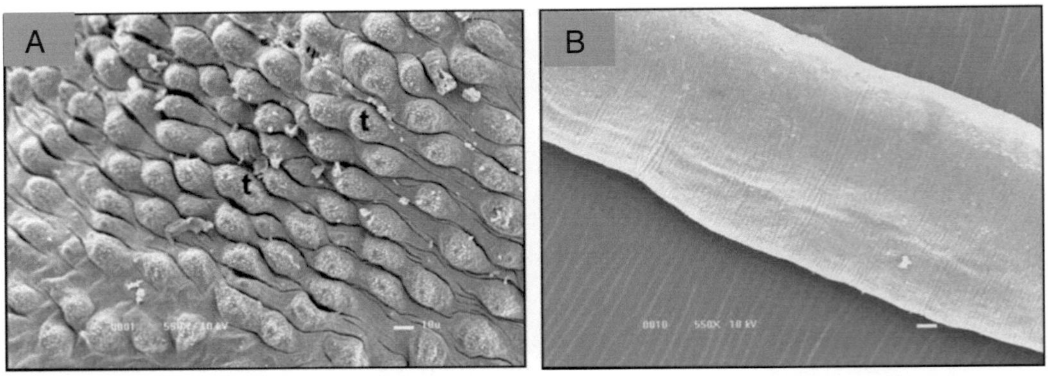

Figure 6. SEM of the tegument of *adult S. mansoni* worms using sodium phosphate buffer. A – tegument of male worm; B – tegument of female worm. **t**: tubercles.

Phosphate Group – Suckers

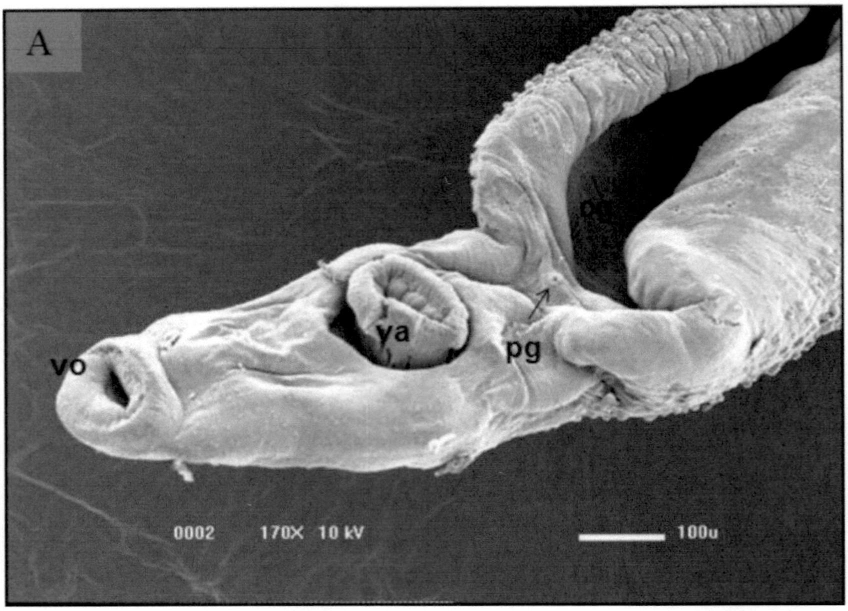

Figure 7. SEM of adult *S. mansoni* worms suckers using sodium phosphate buffer. **A**- male worm, genital pore highlighted (**pg**).

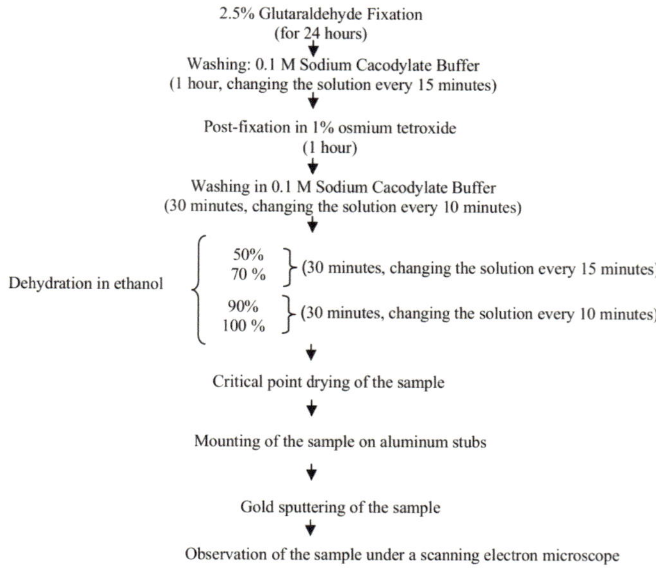

Figure 8. Protocol used by our research group to prepare *S. mansoni* specimens for scanning electron microscopy.

5. Study of the activity of medicinal plants on the tegument of *S. mansoni: Baccharis trimera* (Less) DC, *Cordia verbenacea* DC and *Phyllanthus amarus*

The species *B. trimera, C. verbenacea* and *P. amarus,* whose activity on the tegument of *S. mansoni* was evaluated, are widely used in Brazilian folk medicine. The studied plants were obtained from the Experimental Field of the Chemical, Biological and Agricultural Pluridisciplinary Research Center (CPQBA), Paulínia (22º45'40" S – 47º09'15" W), São Paulo, Brazil. The following fractions were tested, all of them coming from the aerial parts (flowers and/or inflorescences).

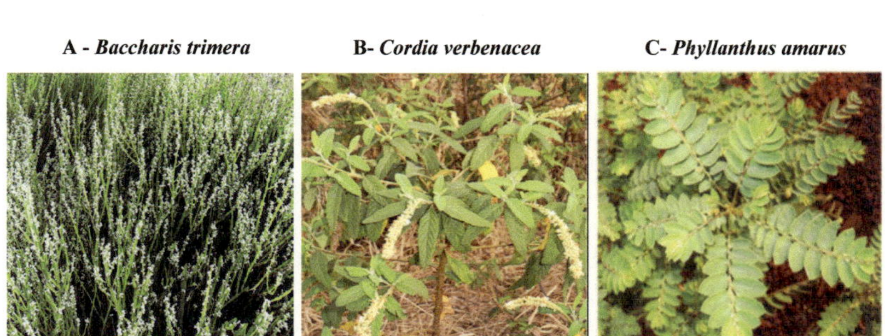

Figure 9. *B. trimera, C. verbenacea* and *P. amarus* specimens. Source: CPQBA, Unicamp, 2011.

- *Baccharis trimera* (Less) DC

The species *B. trimera* (Figure 9-A), known in Brazil as "*carqueja-amarga*", belongs to the family Asteraceae and is used in folk medicine for the treatment of many diseases, in particular hepatic ones. The plant allegedly has tonic, mouth-healing, antipyretic, analgesic, anti-diabetic, and anti-inflammatory properties [75-81]. It is native to the South and Southeast regions of Brazil, also being found in Argentina, Bolivia, Paraguay and Uruguay [82].

B. trimera was used in *in vitro* assays in which mating worms were kept in RPMI-1640 medium with penicillin/streptomycin, incubated in a controlled environment (5% CO_2 and 37°C) [53], and exposed to a fraction hexane fraction, obtained from the fractionation of dichloromethane extract, in lethal concentration of 130 μg/mL for 24 hours. After that period, the worms were prepared for SEM, also according to the protocol shown in Figure 8.

The hexane fraction of *B. trimera* caused changes to the tegument of both males and females and on the oral and ventral suckers. The tegumental peeling was particularly worth noting (Figures 10 to 12).

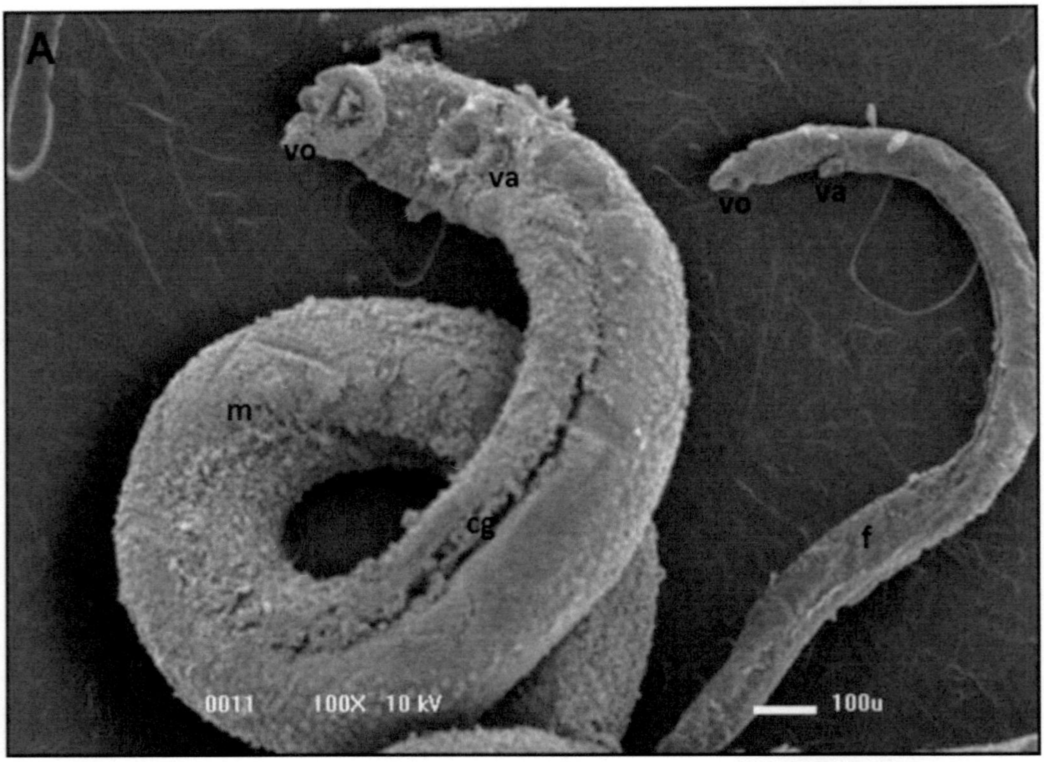

Figure 10. SEM of a *S. mansoni* adult couple after *in vitro* exposure to hexane fraction obtained from the crude dichloromethane extract at the lethal concentration of 130 μg/mL, over an incubation period of 24 hours. **m**- male worm showing changes in its oral **(vo)** and ventral **(va)** suckers, as well as destruction of its tegument; **f –** female worm with tegumental peeling on its body surface.

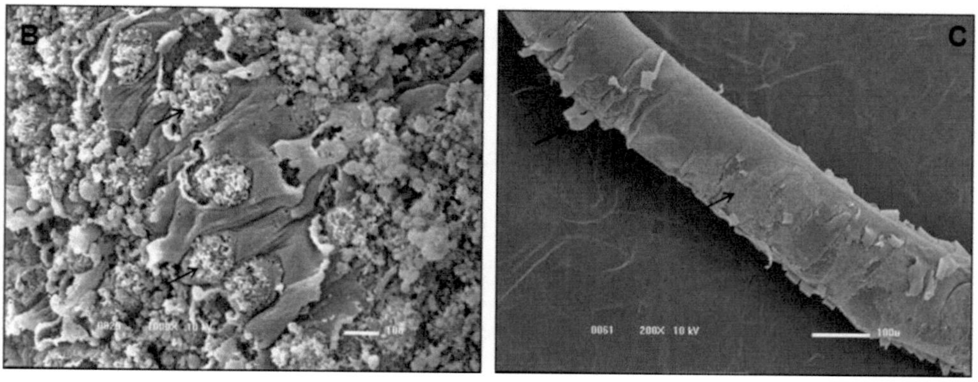

Figure 11. SEM of adult *S. mansoni* specimens after *in vitro* exposure to the hexane fraction obtained from the crude dichloromethane extract at the lethal concentration of 130 µg/mL, over an incubation period of 24 hours. **B.** Male worm, destruction of tubercles and thorns on its tegumental surface. **C.** Female worm with extensive tegumental peeling on its dorsal surface.

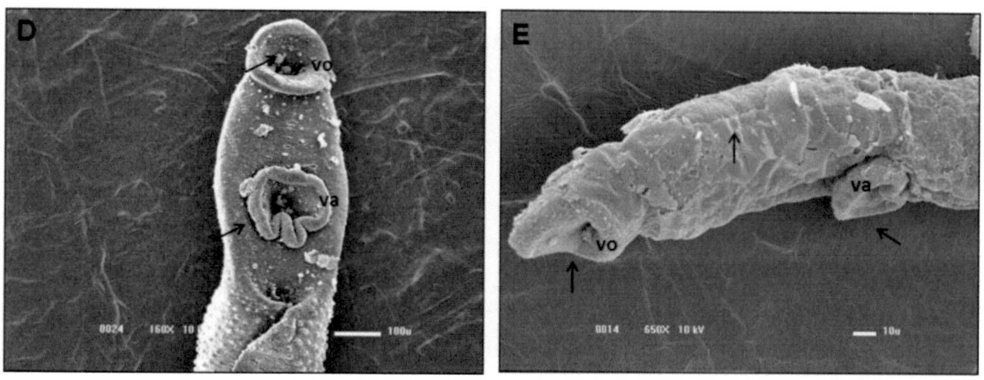

Figure 12. SEM of adult *S. mansoni* specimens after *in vitro* exposure to the hexane fraction obtained from the crude dichloromethane extract at the lethal concentration of 130 µg/mL, over an incubation period of 24 hours. **D.** Male worm with changes in the oral (**vo**) and ventral (**va**) suckers. **E.** Female worm with changes in the suckers and tegumental wrinkling and erosion.

- *Cordia verbenacea* DC

C. verbenacea (Figure 9-B), also referred to as *C. salicina, C. curassavica, C. cylindristachia, Lithocardium fresenii, L. salicinum and L. verbaceum*, is popularly known as *erva-baleeira* or salicina in Brazil. It belongs to the family Boraginaceae and is widely distributed along the Brazilian coast, being found mainly in the littoral zone extending from São Paulo to Santa Catarina [83]. Species of the genus *Cordia* are present in tropical and subtropical areas of Asia, Southern Africa, Australia, Guyana, and South America [84]. Several compounds are found in their aerial parts, including tanins, flavonoids, mucilage, and essential oils. Such parts, along with leaves and inflorescences, have been used in folk medicine in the form of infusions and alcohol extracts because of their antiulcer, antimicrobial and antirheumatic activities, and tonic, analgesic and anti-inflammatory properties [83,85,86]. In view of the variety of chemical groups found in extracts of *C. verbenacea* and their alleged biological properties, that plant is an important material for pharmaceutical research [87].

C. verbenacea were used in *in vivo* assays with mice Balb/c (*Mus musculus*), infected with 70 cercariae of *S. mansoni* (BH strain) by tail immersion [98], and kept in an isolated environment. Forty-five days following infection, the animals were treated orally by esophageal intubation with 300 mg/kg, administered in a single dose, of fraction 3, obtained from the fractionation of the organic fraction, originated from the ethanol extract [99], with a specific concentration of the tested fraction. Fifteen days after treatment, the animals were euthanized by cervical dislocation. The worms were collected by perfusion of the hepatic portal system [100], and washed in 0.9% NaCl solution and subjected to the protocol shown in Figure 8 in order to be analyzed by scanning electron microscopy.

Fraction 3 of *C. verbenacea* caused an erosion on the tegument of both male and female worms. Formation of vesicles and adhesion of host's cells to the surface of worms (Figure 13) were also observed. No damages to the sucker were found.

- *Phyllanthus amarus*

The plants belonging to the genus *Phyllanthus* are widely distributed in most of the tropical and subtropical countries (in both hemispheres) and include between 550 and 750 species. It is believed that around 200 species of that genus are distributed in the Americas, chiefly in the Caribbean and in Brazil [88, 89]. In Brazil, the plants of that genus are popularly known as stonebreaker (*"quebra-pedra"* in Brazilian Portuguese) because they are recognized by their diuretic properties in Brazilian and other countries' folk medicine, being used in the treatment for kidney and bladder disorders. In addition to helping the elimination of kidney stones, they combat intestinal infections, diabetes and hepatitis B [88-90]. The interest in plants of the genus *Phyllanthus* has been considerably increasing, especially for the species *P. amarus* (family Euphorbiaceae) (Figure 9-C), which is scientifically one of the most studied, many of its compounds having already been isolated and chemically identified. *P. amarus* has a long history of usage in folk medicine because of its rich medicinal effects, being reported to possess potent hepatoprotective [91, 92], anti-inflammatory, analgesic [93-94], hypoglycaemic [95], antiplasmodial (against *Plasmodium berghei*) [96], and antioxidant [97] properties.

P. amarus were used in *in vivo* assays with mice Balb/c (*Mus musculus*), infected with 70 cercariae of *S. mansoni* (BH strain) by tail immersion [98], and kept in an isolated environment. Forty-five days following infection, the animals were treated orally by esophageal intubation [99], with the butanolic fraction 2 in the concentration of the 100 mg/kg for three days. Fifteen days after treatment, the animals were euthanized by cervical dislocation. The worms were collected by perfusion of the hepatic portal system [100], washed in 0.9% NaCl solution and subjected to the protocol shown in Figure 8 in order to be analyzed by scanning electron microscopy.

The butanolic fraction 2 of *P. amarus* caused damage to the male worms' tegument, including perforations, changes in the tubercles, peeling, and formation of vesicles and protuberances. Contraction and swelling were noticed in the region around the suckers (Figure 14). No damage were found in the tegument of females. This fraction did not cause the separation of coupled worms, thus female worms remained in the gynaecophoric canal protected from the action of the butanolic fraction 2.

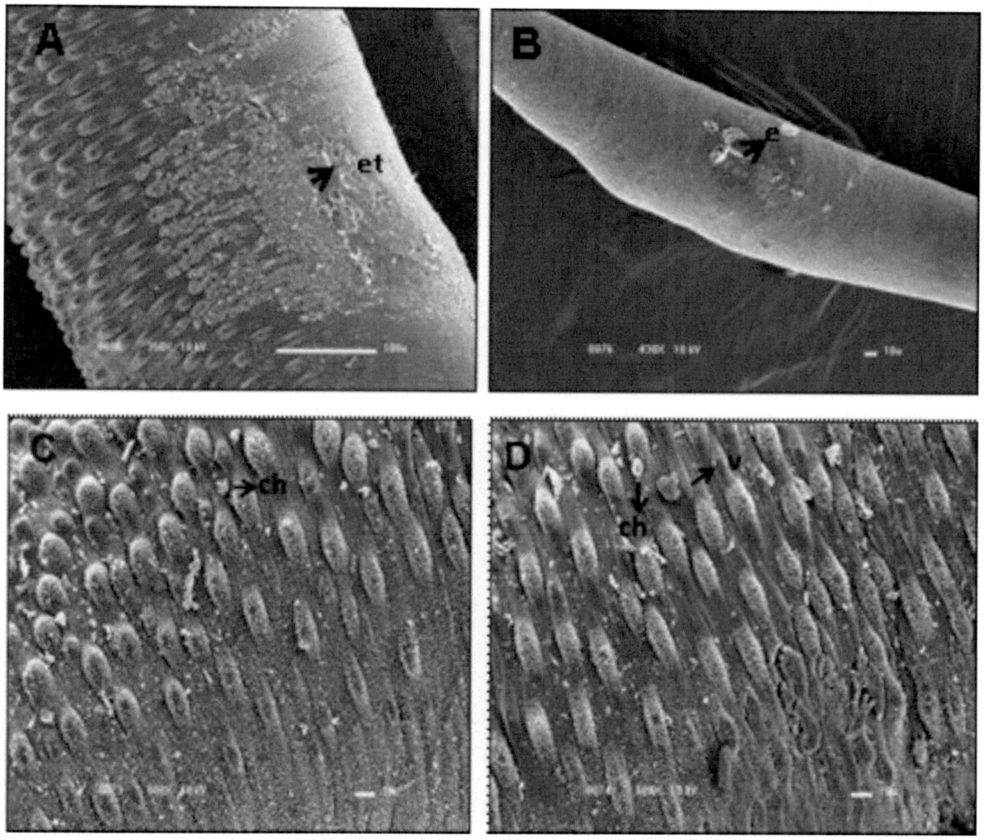

Figure 13. SEM of adult *S. mansoni* specimens after *in vivo* assay with fraction 3 obtained from the organic fraction of *C. verbenacea* at the concentration of 300 mg/kg. **A-B.** Male and female worms, respectively, showing peeling of the tegument. **C-D.** Male worms showing adhesion of host's cells to its tegument and formation of vesicles. **et** – erosion of the tegument; **ch** – host's cells adhered to the surface of *S. mansoni*; **l** – host's leukocytes; **dt** – destruction of the tegument; **v** – vesicle.

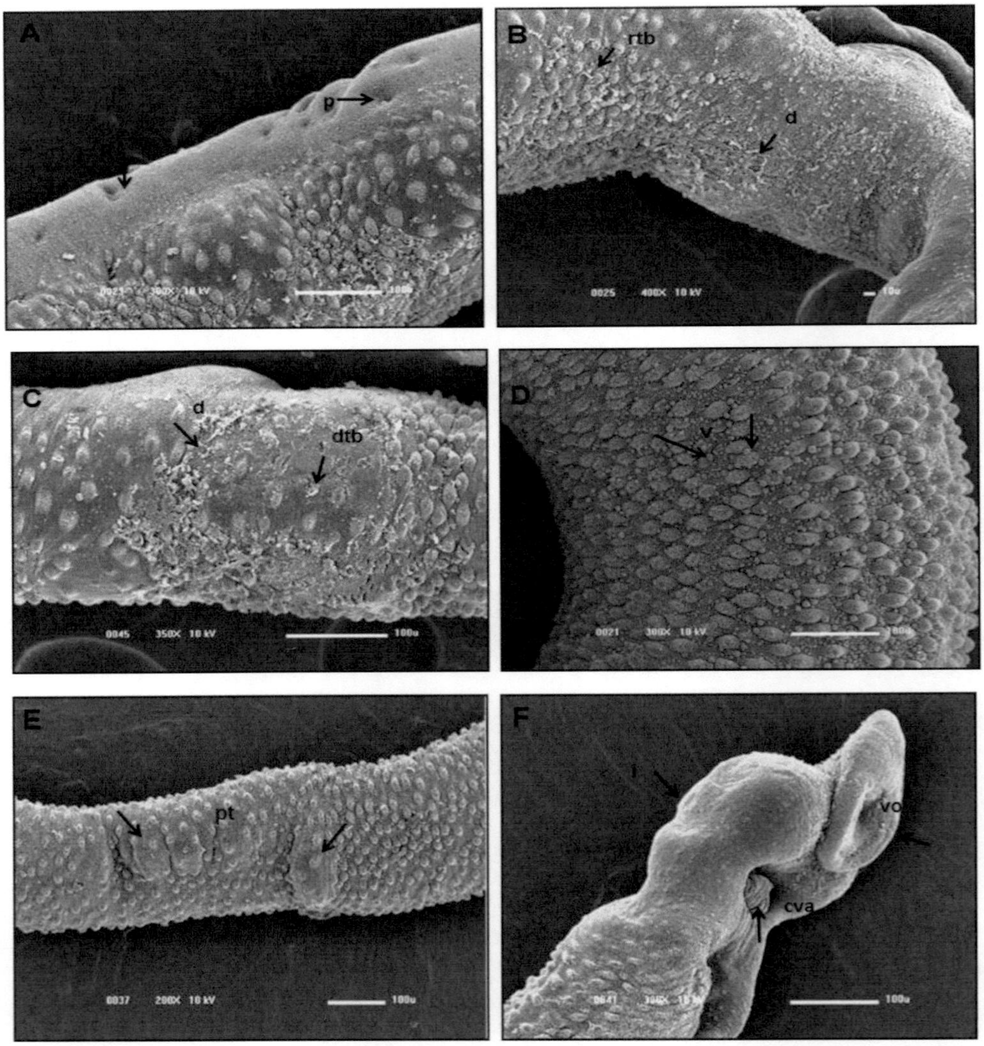

Figure 14. SEM of adult *S. mansoni* specimens after *in vivo* assay with butane fraction 2 from butane extract at the concentration of 100 mg/kg/3 consecutive days. **A.** Area of the gynaecophoric canal showing perforations (**p**). **B.** Rupture of tubercles (**rtb**) and peeling (**d**) on the tegument of a male worm. **C.** Peeling (**d**) and destruction of tubercles (**dtb**). **D.** Formation of several vesicles (**v**). **E.** Formation of protuberances (**pt**) on the tegument. **F.** Contraction of the ventral sucker (**cvv**) and swelling (**i**) of the region around the suckers.

6. Conclusions

- The combined use of 0.1 M sodium cacodylate buffer and 2.5% glutaraldehyde and the reduction in fixation time provided more distinct images with no artefacts, in contrary to the combination of Karnovsky solution with 0.1 M phosphate buffer.

- The tested fractions of *B. trimera, C. verbenacea* and *P. amarus* caused tegumental changes in adult *S. mansoni* specimens, including peeling or erosion of the surface membrane, formation of vesicles, destruction of tubercles, and modifications in the suckers. It is worth noting that such changes were more intense in male worms.

- Since the tegument of *S. mansoni* is a major chemotherapeutic target, we can infer that the fractions of *B. trimera, C. verbenacea* and *P. amarus* have a promising schistosomicidal activity, more studies being needed in order to isolate and identify their compounds active against the worm and to understand their mechanism of action on the tegument.

Acknowledgments

The authors are thankful to CAPES and FAPESP for financial support.

Author details

Claudineide Nascimento Fernandes de Oliveira[1*], Rosimeire Nunes de Oliveira[1], Tarsila Ferraz Frezza[1], Vera Lúcia Garcia Rehder[2] and Silmara Marques Allegretti[1]

*Address all correspondence to: claudineide@gmail.com

1 Department of Animal Biology, State University of Campinas (Unicamp), Campinas, São Paulo, Brazil

2 Division of Organic Chemistry and Pharmaceuticals, Chemical, Biological and Agricultural Pluridisciplinary Research Center (CPQBA), Paulínia, São Paulo, Brazil

References

[1] Engels D, Chitsulo L, Montresor A, Savioli L. The global epidemiological situation of schistosomiasis and new approaches to control and research. Acta Tropica 2002; 82: 139-146.

[2] Steinmann P, Keiser J, Bos R, Tanner M, Utzinger J. Schistosomiais and water resources development: systematic review, meta-analysis, and estimates of people at risk. The Lancet Infectious Diseases 2006; 6: 411-425.

[3] Bina JC, Prata A. Esquistossomose na área hiperendêmica de Taquarendi. I – Infecção pelo *Schistosoma mansoni* e formas graves. Revista da Sociedade Brasileira de Medicina Tropical 2003; 36: 211-6.

[4] World Health Organization. World health report 2004: changing history. Geneva: WHO; 2004.

[5] Lambertucci JR. Acute schistosomiasis mansoni: revisited and reconsidered. Memórias Instituto Oswaldo Cruz 2010; 105: 422-435.

[6] World Health Organization. Media Centre - Factsheets n°115 - Schistosomiasis. http://www.who.int/mediacentre/factsheets/fs115/en/index.html (accessed 18 August 2012).

[7] Parise-Filho R, Silveira MAB. Panorama atual da esquistossomíase no mundo. Brazilian Journal of Pharmaceutical Sciences 2001; 37: 123-135.

[8] Anaruma FF, SANTOS R. F. Indicadores da relação entre estrutura da paisagem, degradação ambiental e esquistossomose mansoni. Anais do VIII Congresso de Ecologia do Brasil: September 23- 28, 2007, Caxambu – Minas Gerais - Brazil.

[9] Cardim, LL, Ferraudo AS, Pacheco STA, Reis RB, Silva MMN, CARNEIRO DDMT, Bavia ME. Identifi cation of schistosomiasis risk areas using spatial analysis in Lauro de Freitas, Bahia State, Brazil. Caderno de Saúde Pública 2011; 27(5): 899-908.

[10] Departamento de Vigilância Epidemiológica, Secretaria de Vigilância em Saúde, Ministério da Saúde. Guia de vigilância epidemiológica. 7a Ed. Brasília: Ministério da Saúde; 2009.

[11] Galvão AF. Impacto do tratamento com praziquantel na infecção por *Schistosoma mansoni* em adolescentes do município de São Lourenço da Mata, área endêmica da esquistossomose em Pernambuco / Impact of treatment with praziquantel on *Schistosoma mansoni* infection in adolescents from the municipality of São Lourenço da Mata, an endemic area of schistosomiasis in Pernambuco. PhD thesis. Instituto Oswaldo Cruz; 2010.

[12] Katz N. Terapêutica experimental da esquistossomose mansoni, In: Carvalho OS, Coelho PMZ, Lenzi HL. (eds.) *Schistosoma mansoni* & esquistossomose uma visão multidisciplinar. Rio de Janeiro - Brazil: Fiocruz; 2008. p 825-870.

[13] Utzinger J, Chollet J, Tu ZW, Xiao SH, Tanner M. Comparative study of the effects of artemether and artesunate on juvenile and adult *Schistosoma mansoni* in experimentally infected mice. Transactions of the Royal Society of Tropical Medicine and Hygiene 2002; 96: 318-323.

[14] Shaohong L, Kumagai T, Qinghua A, Xiaolan Y, Ohmae H, Yabu Y, Siwen L, Liyong W, Maruyama H, Ohta N. Evaluation of the antihelmintic effects of artesunate against experimental *Schistosoma mansoni* infection in mice using different treatment protocols. Parasitology International 2006; 55: 63-68.

[15] Fallon PG, Doenhoff MJ. Drug-resistant schistosomiasis: resistance topraziquantel and oxamniquine induced in *Schistosoma mansoni* in mice is drug specific. American Journal of Tropical Medicine and Hygiene 1994; 53: 61-62.

[16] Pica-Mattoccia L, Cioli D. Sex and stage-related sensitivity of *Schistosoma mansoni* to *in vivo* and *in vitro* praziquantel treatment. International Journal for Parasitology 2004; 34: 527-533.

[17] Doenhoff MJ, Cioli D, Utzinger J. Praziquantel: mechanism of action, resistance and new derivatives for schistosomiasis. Current Opinion in Infectious Diseases 2008; 21: 659-667.

[18] Ministério da Saúde. Política nacional de plantas medicinais e fitoterápicos - Série B - Textos básicos de saúde. Brasília – Brazil: Ministério da Saúde; 2006.

[19] Garcia ES, Silva ACP, Gilbert B, Santos RR, Tomasi, T. Fitoterápicos. Campinas – Brazil: André Tosello; 1996.

[20] Shaw MK, Erasmus DA. *Schistosoma mansoni*: praziquantel-induced changes to the female reproductive system. Experimental Parasitology 1988; 65: 31-42.

[21] Bertão HG, Silva RAR, Padilha RJR, Albuquerque MCPA, Rádis-Baptista G. Ultrastructural analysis of miltefosine-induced surface membrane damage in adult *Schistosoma mansoni* BH strain worms. Parasitology Research 2012; 110(6) 2465-2473.

[22] Lima CMBL. Investigação da atividade antiparasitária do *Allium sativum* L. *in vitro* e *in vivo*. PhD thesis. Laboratório de tecnologia farmacêutica UFPB, João Pessoa-PB; 2011.

[23] Reda ES, Ouhtit A, Abdeen SH, El-Shabasy EA. Structural changes of *Schistosoma mansoni* adult worms recovered from C57BL/6 mice treated with radiation-attenuated vaccine and/or praziquantel against infection. Parasitology Research 2012; 110(2) 979-992.

[24] Shuhua X, Binggui S, Chollet J, Utzinger J, Tanner M. Tegumental changes in adult *Schistosoma mansoni* harbored in mice treated with artemether. The Journal of Parasitology 2000; 86: 1125-1132.

[25] Skelly PJ, Wilson RA. Making sense of the schistosome surface. Advances in Parasitology 2006; 65: 185:284.

[26] Van Hellemon JJ, Retra K, Brouwers JF, Van Balkom BW, Yazdanbakhsh M, Shoemaker CB, Tielens AG. Functions of the tegument of schistosomes: clues from the proteome and lipidome. International Journal for Parasitology 2006; 36: 691-699.

[27] Moraes J. 2012. Antischistosomal natural compounds: present challenges for new drug screens. In: Rodriguez-Morales (ed.) Current topics in tropical medicine. Rijeka: InTech Open; 2012. p 333-358. Available from http://cdn.intechopen.com/pdfs/32504/InTech-Antischistosomal_natural_compounds_present_challenges_for_new_drug_screens.pdf (accessed 18 september 2012).

[28] Gonnert R. Uber rudimentare weibliche Geschlechtsanlagen bei Bilharzia mansoni-Mannchen. Zeitschrift für Tropenmedizin und Parasitologie 1949; 1: 272-279.

[29] Gönnert R. Schistosomiasis studies. II. Übedie Eibildung bei *Schistosoma mansoni* und das Schicksal der Eier Wirtsorganismus. Zeitschrift für Tropenmedizin und Parasitologie 1955; 6: 33-52

[30] Senft AW. A perfusion apparatus for maintenance and observation of schistosomes *in vitro.* Journal of Parasitology 1959; 44: 652-658.

[31] Hockley DJ. Small spines on the egg shells of *Schistosoma.* Parasitology 1968; 58: 367-370.

[32] Senft AW, Gibler WB. *Schistosoma mansoni* tegumental appendages: scanning microscopy following thiocarbohydrazide-osmium preparation. American Journal of Tropical Medicine and Hygiene 1977; 26(6 Pt 1) 1169-77.

[33] Hockley DJ, McLaren DJ. *Schistosoma mansoni*: Changes in the outer membrane of the tegument during development from cercaria to adult worm. International Journal for Parasitology 1973; 3: 13-20.

[34] Becker B, Mehlhorn H, Andrews P, Eckert J. Light and electron microscopic studies on the effect of praziquantel on *Schistosoma mansoni, Dicrocoelium dendriticum* and *Fasciola hepatica* (Trematoda) *in vivo*. Parasitology Research 1980; 63: 113-128.

[35] Kohn A, López-Alvarez ML, Katz N. Transmission and scanning electron microscopical studies in the tegument of male Schistosoma mansoni after oxamniquine treatment. Annales de Parasitologie Humaine et Comparée 1982; 57: 285-291.

[36] Magalhães-Filho A; Melo MEB, Padovan PA, Padovan PP. Schistosoma mansoni: structural damage after treatment with oxamniquine. Memórias do Instituto Oswaldo Cruz 1987; 82: 347-352.

[37] Shaw MK, Erasmus DA. *Schistosoma mansoni:* dose-related tegumental changes after *in vivo* treatment with praziquantel. Parasitology Research 1983; 69:643-653.

[38] Doenhoff MJ, Sabah AA, Fletcher C, Webbe G, Bain J. Evidence for a immune-dependent action of praziquantel on *Schistosoma mansoni* in mice. Transactions of the Royal Society of Tropical Medicine and Hygiene 1987; 81: 947-951.

[39] Brindley PJ, Strand M, Norden AP, Sher A. Role of host antibody in the chemotherapeutic action of praziquantel against *Schistosoma mansoni:* identification of target antigens. Molecular and Biochemical Parasitology 1989; 34: 99-108.

[40] Brickes CS, Depenbusch JW, Benett JL, Thompson DF. The relationship between tegumental disruption and muscle contraction in *Schistosoma mansoni* exposed to various compounds. Parasitology Research 1983; 69: 61-67.

[41] Albuquerque MCPA, Pitta MGR, Irmão JI, Peixoto CA, Malagueño E, Santana JV, Lima MCA, Galdino SL, Pitta IR. Tegumental Alterations in Adult *Schistosoma mansoni* Treated with Imidazolidine Derivatives. Latin America Journal of Pharmacy 2007; 26: 65-9

[42] Manneck T, Haggenmüller Y, Keiser J. Morphological effects and tegumental alterations induced by mefloquine on schistosomula and adult flukes of *Schistosoma mansoni.* Parasitology 2010; 137: 85-98

[43] Xiao S, Xue J, Shen B. 2010 Transmission electron microscopic observation on ultrastructural alterations in *Schistosoma japonicum* caused by mefloquine. Parasitology Research 2010; 106(5): 1179-1187.

[44] El Ridi R, Aboueldahab M, Tallima H, Salah M, Mahana N, Fawzi S, Mohamed SH, Fahmy OM. *In vitro* and *in vivo* activities of arachidonic acid against *Schistosoma mansoni* and *Schistosoma haematobium*. Antimicrobial Agents and Chemotherapy 2010; 54: 3383-3389.

[45] Abdul-Ghani R, Loutfy N, Sheta M, Hassan A. Artemether shows promising female schistosomicidal and ovicidal effects on the Egyptian strain of *Schistosoma mansoni* after maturity of infection. Parasitology Research 2011; 108(5) 1199-1205.

[46] Oliveira RN, Rehder VLG, Oliveira ASS, Montarinari-Júnior I, Carvalho JE, Ruiz ALTG, Jeraldo VLS, Linhares AX, Allegretti SM. *Schistosoma mansoni*: *In vitro* schistosomicidal activity of essential oil of *Baccharis trimera* (less) DC. Experimental Parasitology 2012; 132(2) 135-143.

[47] Minsky M, inventor. Microscopy Apparatus. US Pat. n. 3,013,467, 1961 Dec. 19.

[48] Egger MD, Petran M. New reflected-light microscope for viewing unstained brain and ganglion Cells. Science 1967; 157: 305-307.

[49] Minsky M. Memoir on Inventing the Confocal Scanning Microscopy. Scanning 1988; 10: 128-138.

[50] Davidovits P, Egger MD. Photomicrography of Corneal Endothelial Cells *in vivo.* Nature 1973; 244: 366-367.

[51] Moraes J, Nascimento C, Lopes POMV, Nakano E, Yamaguchi LF, Kato MJ, Kawano T. *Schistosoma mansoni*: *In vitro schistosomicidal activity* of *piplartine.* Experimental Parasitology 2011; 127(2) 357-364.

[52] Magalhães LG, Kapadia GJ, Tonuci LRS, Caixeta SC, Parreira NA, Rodrigues V, Silva-Filho AA. In vitro schistosomicidal effects of some phloroglucinol derivatives from *Dryopteris* species against *Schistosoma mansoni* adult worms. Parasitology Research 2010; 106: 395–401

[53] Xiao SH, Keiser J, Chollet J, Utzinger J, Dong Y, Endriss Y, Vennerstrom JL, Tanner M. . *In vitro* and *in vivo* activities of synthetic trioxolanes against major human schistosome species. Antimicrobial Agents and Chemotherapy 2007; 51: 1440–1445.

[54] Braguine CG, Costa ES, Magalhães LG, Rodrigues V, Da Silva Filho AA, Bastos JK, Silva ML, Cunha WR, Januário AH, Pauletti PM. Schistosomicidal evaluation of *Zanthoxylum naranjillo* and its isolated compounds against *Schistosoma mansoni* adult worms. Zeitschrift für Naturforschung 2009; 64: 793-797.

[55] Magalhães LG, Machado CB, Morais ER, Moreira EBC, Soares CS, Silva SH, Da Silva Filho AA, Rodrigues V. *In vitro* schistosomicidal activity of curcumin against *Schistosoma mansoni* adult worms. Parasitology Research 2009; 104: 1197-1201.

[56] Neves JK, Botelho SP, Melo CM, Pereira VR, Lima, MC, Pitta IR, Albuquerque MC, Galdino SL. Biological and immunological activity of new imidazolidines against adult worms of *Schistosoma mansoni.* Parasitology Research 2010; 107: 531-538.

[57] Melo NI, Magalhães LG, Carvalho CE, Wakabayashi KAL, Aguiar GP, Ramos RC, Mantovani ALL, Turatti ICC, Rodrigues V, Groppo M, Cunha WR, Veneziani RCS, Crotti AEM. Schistosomicidal Activity of the Essential Oil of *Ageratum conyzoides* L. (Asteraceae) against Adult *Schistosoma mansoni* Worms. Molecules 2011; 16: 762-773.

[58] Portela J, Boissier J, Gourbal B, Pradines V, Collière V, Coslédan F, Meunier B, Robert A. Antischistosomal Activity of Trioxaquines: *In Vivo* Efficacy and Mechanism of Action on *Schistosoma mansoni,* PLOS Neglected Tropical Disease 2012; 6(2): 1474.

[59] Shuhua X, Binggui S, Utzinger J, Chollet J, Tanner M. *Transmission* electron microscopic observations on ultrastructural damage in juvenile *Schistosoma mansoni* caused by artemether. Acta Tropica 2002; 81: 53–61

[60] Castro LAS. Processamento de Amostras para Microscopia Eletrônica de Varredura – documentos 93. Pelotas – Brazil: Embrapa; 2002.

[61] Dedavid BA, Gomes CI, Machado G. Microscopia Eletrônica de Varredura - Aplicação e Preparação de Amostras – Materiais poliméricos, metálicos e semicondutores. Porto Alegre - Brazil: EDPUCRS; 2007.

[62] Ploem JS. "Laser scanning fluorescence microscopy," Applied Optics 1987; 26: 3226-3231.

[63] Claxton NS, Fellers TJ, Davidson MW. 2006. Laser scanning confocal microscopy. Department of Optical Microscopy and Digital Imaging, National High Magnetic Field Laboratory, The Florida State University http://www.olympusfluoview.com/theory/LSCMIntro.pdf. (accessed 18 August 2012).

[64] Silveira M. 1998. Preparo de amostras biológicas para microscopia eletrônica de varredura. In: SOUZA W. Técnicas básicas de microscopia eletrônica aplicada às ciências biológicas. Rio de Janeiro - Brazil: Departamento de editoração eletrônica da UENF. p33-44.

[65] Magalhães-Filho A, Melo MEB, Padovan PA, PADOVAN IP. *Schistosoma mansoni:* estructural damage after treatment with oxamniquine. Memórias do Instituto Oswaldo Cruz 1987; 82(Suppl. IV): 347-352.

[66] *Voge M, Bueding E. Schistosoma mansoni:* Tegumental surface alterations induced by subcurative doses of the schistosomicide amoscanate. Experimental Parasitology 1980; 50(2) 251-259.

[67] Mohamed SH. Scanning electron microscopical studies on the tegument of adult worms of *Schistosoma mansoni* originating from ultraviolet-irradiated and non-irradiated cercariae. Journal of. Helminthology 1999; 73: 157-161.

[68] Miller FH, Tulloch Jr SG, Kuntz RE. Scanning electron microscopy of integumental surface of *Schistosoma mansoni.* Journal of Parasitology 1972; 58(4) 693-698.

[69] Kuntz RE, Tulloch GS, Davidson DL, Huang T. Scanning electron microscopy of the integumental surfaces of *Schistosoma haematobium.* Journal of Parasitology 1976; 65: 63-69.

[70] Caulfield JP, Korman G, Butterworth AE, Hogan M, David JR. The Adherence of Human Neutrophils and Eosinophils to Schistosomula: Evidence for Membrane Fusion between Cells and Parasites. The Journal of Cell Biology 1980; 86: 46-63.

[71] Fried B, Graczyk TK, editors Advances in Trematode Biology, New York: CRC Press Ed.; 1997.

[72] Lima CMBL, Freitas FIS, Morais LCSL, Cavalcanti MGS, Ferreira da Silva L, Padilha RJR, Barbosa CGS, Santos FAB, Alves LC, Diniz MFFM. Ultrastructural study on the morphological changes to male worms of *Schistosoma mansoni* after *in vitro* exposure to allicin. Revista da Sociedade Brasileira de Medicina Tropical 2011; 44(3):327-330.

[73] Sesso A. Fixação de sistemas biológicos. In: Souza W (ed.) Técnicas básicas de microscopia eletrônica aplicada às ciências biológicas. Rio de Janeiro: Departamento de editoração eletrônica da UENF;1998. p1-17.

[74] Padron TS. Soluções tampões.. In: Souza W (ed.) Técnicas básicas de microscopia eletrônica aplicada às ciências biológicas. Rio de Janeiro: Departamento de editoração eletrônica da UENF; 1998. p18-21.

[75] Borella JC, Duarte DP, Novaretti AAG, Menezes JRA, França SC, Rufato CB, Santos PAS, Veneziani RCS, Lopes NP. Variabilidade sazonal do teor de saponinas de *Baccharis trimera* (Less.) DC (Carqueja) e isolamento de flavona. Revista Brasileira de Farmacognosia 2006; 16(4) 557-561.

[76] Corrêa MP. Dicionário das Plantas Úteis do Brasil e das Exóticas Cultivadas. Rio de Janeiro – Brazil: Imprensa Nacional; 1984.

[77] Fukuda M, Ohkoshi E, Makino M, Fujimoto Y. Studies on the constituents of the leaves of *Baccharis dracunculifolia* (Asteraceae) and their cytotoxic activity. Chemical Pharmaceutical Bulletin 2006; 54: 1465–1468.

[78] Gené R.M., Cartarana C, Adzet T, Marin E, Parella T, Canigueral S. Anti-inflammatory and analgesic activity of *Baccharis trimera*: identification of its active constituents. Planta Médica 1996; 62(3) 232-235.

[79] Moreira FPM, Coutinho V, Montanher ABP, Caro MSB, Brighente IMC, Pizzolatti MG. Flavonóides e triterpenos de *Baccharis eudotenuifolia* - Bioatividade sobre *Artemisia salina*. Química Nova 2003; 26: 309-311.

[80] Torres LM, Gamberini MT, Roque NF, Lima-Landman MT, Souccar C, Lapa AJ. Diterpene from *Baccharis trimera* with a relaxant effect on rat vascular smooth muscle. Phytochemistry 2000; 55: 617–619.

[81] Verdi LG, Brighent IMC, Pizzolatti MG. Gênero *Baccharis* (Asteraceae): Aspectos químicos, econômicos e biológicos. Química Nova 2005; 28: 85–94.

[82] Bona CM, Biasi LA, Zanette F, Nakashima T. Propagation of three speciesof Baccharis by cuttings. Revista Ciência Rural 2005; 35: 223–226.

[83] Carvalho Jr PM, Rodrigues RF, Sawaya AC, Marques MO, Shimizu MT. Chemical composition and antimicrobial activity of the essential oil of *Cordia verbenacea* D.C. Journal of Ethnopharmacology 2004; 95(2-3) 297–301.

[84] Ficarra R, Ficarra P, Tommasini S. Leaf extracts of some Cordia species analgesic and anti-inflammatory activities as well as their chromatographic analysis. Farmaco 1995; 50(4) 245-256.

[85] Sertié JAA, Woisky RG, Wiezel G., Rodrigues M. Pharmacological assay of *Cordia verbenacea* V: oral and topical anti-inflammatory activity, analgesic effect and fetus toxicity of a crude leaf extract. Phytomedicine 2005; 12(5) 338-344.

[86] Passos GF, Fernandes ES, Cunha FM, Ferreira J, Pianowski LF, Campos MM, Campos MM, Calixto JB.. Anti-inflammatory and anti-allergic properties of the essential oil and active compounds from *Cordia verbenacea*. Journal of Ethnopharmacololy 2006; 110(2) 323–333.

[87] Michielin EMZ, Salvador AA, Riehl CAS, Smânia-Jr A, Smânia EFA, Ferreira SRS. Chemical composition and antibacterial activity of *Cordia verbenacea* extracts obtained by different methods. Bioresource Technology 2009; 100(24) 6615-6623.

[88] Calixto JB, Santos AR, Cechinel-Filho V, Yunes RA. A review of the plants of the 44 genus *Phyllanthus*: their chemistry, pharmacology, and therapeutic potential. Medicinal Research Reviews 1998; 18(4) 225–258.

[89] Torres DSC, Cordeiro I, Giulietti AM. O Gênero *Phyllanthus* L. (*Euphorbiaceae)* na Chapada Diamantina, Bahia, Brasil. Acta Botanica Brasilica 2003; 17(2) 265-278.

[90] Khatoon S, Rai V, Rawat AKSR, Mehrota S. Comparative pharmacognostic studies of three *Phyllanthus* species. *Journal of Ethnopharmacology* 2006; 104(1-2) 79-86.

[91] Krithika R, Mohankumar R, Verma RJ, Shrivastav PS, Mohamed IL, Gunasekaran P, Narasimhan S. Isolation, characterization and antioxidative effect of phyllanthin against CCl4-induced toxicity in HepG2 cell line. Chemico-Biological Interactions 2009, 181: 351-358.

[92] Pramyothin P, Ngamtin C, Poungshompoo S, Chaichantipyuth C. Hepatoprotective activity of *Phyllantus amarus* Schum. et. Thonn. Extract in ethanol treated rats: *In vitro* and *in vivo* studies. Journal of Ethnopharmacology 2007; 114(2) 169-173.

[93] Kassuya CA, Rehder VLG, Melo LV, Silvestre AA, Calixto JB. Anti-inflammatory properties of extracts, fractions and lignans isolated from *Phyllanthus amarus*. Planta Medica 2005; 71(8) 721-726.

[94] Kassuya CA, Silvestre AA, Menezes de Lima O, Marotta Jr DM, Rehder VLG, Calixto JB. Anti-inflammatory and antiallodynic actions of the lignin niranthin isolated from *Phyllanthus amarus* evidence for interaction with platelet activating factor receptor. European Journal of Pharmacology 2006; 546(1-3) 182-188.

[95] Raphael KR, Sabu MC, Kuttan R. Hypoglycemic effect of methanol extract of *Phyllanthus amarus* Schumach and Thonn on alloxan induced *diabetes mellitus* in rats and its relation with antioxidant potential. Indian Journal of Experimental Biology 2002, 40(8) 905-909.

[96] Dapper DV, Aziagba BN, Ebong OO. Antiplasmodial effects of the aqueous extract of *Phyllanthus amarus* Schumach and Thonn against *Plasmodium berghei* in Swiss albino mice. Nigerian Journal of Physiological Sciences 2007; 22(1-2) 19-25.

[97] Karuna R, Reddy SS, Baskar R, Saralakumari D. Antioxidant potential of aqueous extract of *Phyllanthus amarus* in rats. Indian Journal of Pharmacology 2009; 41(2) 64-67.

[98] Olivier L, Stirewalt A. An efficient method for exposure of mice to cercariae of *Schistosoma mansoni.* Journal of Parasitology 1952; 38: 19-23.

[99] Delgado VS, Suárez DP, Cesari IM, Hincan RN. Experimental chemotherapy of *Schistosoma mansoni* with praziquantel and oxamniquine: differential effect of single or combined formulations of drugs on various strains and on both sexes of the parasite. Parasitology Research 1992; 78: 648-654.

[100] YollesTK, Moore PV, De Ginsti DL, Ripson CA, Meleney HE. A technique for the perfusion of laboratory animals for the recovery of schistosomes. Journal of Parasitology 1947; 33: 419-26.

Chapter 9

Solving the Riddle of the Lung-Stage Schistosomula Paved the Way to a Novel Remedy and an Efficacious Vaccine for Schistosomiasis

Rashika El Ridi and Hatem Tallima

Additional information is available at the end of the chapter

http://dx.doi.org/10.5772/52922

1. Introduction

The field of schistosomiasis vaccine has suffered from several entrenched dogmas, which have delayed progress.

The first dogma states that the main mechanism of innate and acquired immunity-related parasite attrition is antibody-dependent cell-mediated cytotoxicity (ADCC). ADCC has been shown to effectively mediate killing of 3-, 18- or 24 hr-old schistosomula in human, mouse, and rat models. However, this phenomenon is of no in vivo relevance as larvae of this age are still in the epidermis, impervious to host immune attacks. Intact, healthy older larvae, pre-adults and adult schistosomes are entirely invisible to the immune system, and thus, are never threatened by ADCC in vitro or in vivo. Concurrently, the immune effectors "hunt" for larvae in the pulmonary capillaries, proposed by von Lichtenberg et al. in 1977 [1] as a plausible mechanism for resistance to infection, was entirely neglected, and never mentioned or referred to.

Second dogma is to consider parasite surface membrane antigens of great importance as vaccine antigens, because they reside at the host-parasite interface, and were shown to induce robust immune responses. However, schistosome surface membrane molecules are hidden, inaccessible to host antibodies, and accordingly, induced immune effectors are unable to interact with the parasite.

Third, stressing that Th1 immune responses are the pillars for acquired immunity to larval infection in mice. This dogma is entrenched notwithstanding the numerous reports documenting the importance of exclusive type 2 immune responses in rat, monkey, and human schistosomiasis, and despite that larval antigens induce principally Th1 related cytokines and antibodies that are not entirely protective in mice. Enhancement of these Th1 responses during mouse immunization, via the use of Th1-biased constructs and adjuvants, consistently elicited only partial resistance, with candidate vaccine antigens discarded one after the other.

This review aims to dispel these dogmas and opens a new avenue for the development of a remedy and vaccine for schistosomiasis.

2. Body

2.1. Schistosomiasis

Schistosomiasis, also known as bilharziosis, bilharzia, or snail fever, is endemic in 74 countries of the Developing World, infecting between 391 and 600 million people worldwide. with close to 800 million, mostly children, at risk [2,3]. The disease burden is estimated to exceed 70 million disability-adjusted life-years [4]. The causative agents are flatworms, dioecious (separate sex) trematodes, of the family Schistosomatidae, with *Schistosoma mansoni* and *Schistosoma haematobium* responsible for the largest numbers of human infections. The infective stage, the cercaria, invades host skin, and stays in the blood- and lymph-free epidermis for a minimum of 40 and up to 72 hr, impervious to innate immunity effectors [5,6]. The parasite develops into a schistosomulum, exchanging the classical outer membrane for a double lipid bilayer covering [7], and releasing in the process of physiological and biochemical changes numerous enzymes and other molecules, which may interact with the innate immunity receptors on keratinocytes and Langerhans cells [4,8-11]. The innate immunity cells proceed to activation of the acquired immune system, and produce cytokines that shape the amount and direction of the adaptive immune responses to the developing parasite [4,8-10]. Schistosomula then penetrate dermal blood vessels, and remain intravascular for their life span, and therefore, schistosomes of the genus *Schistosoma* are known as blood flukes [12]. The schistosomula travel via the pulmonary artery reaching the lungs within 4-6 and 6-10 days for *S. mansoni* and *S. haematobium*, respectively [13], painstakingly negociate the lung capillaries, then migrate to the hepatic portal vessels, where they start to actively feed, mature, and copulate. It is important here to recall that developing (and mature) schistosomes live in the blood vessels and capillaries, and hence, released, excreted, or secreted molecules are blood-borne products, which likely access macrophages, dendritic cells, and B cells in the spleen rather than the lung tissue draining lymph nodes. It is documented that developing schistosomula products elicit predominant T helper (Th) Th1 and Th17 immune responses, dominated by interferon-gamma (IFN-g) and interleukin (IL)-17, and IgG2a and IgG2b antibodies [14-19]. The male carrying the female in the gynaecophoric groove, the schist, then migrates to the mesenteric venules (*S. mansoni*) or the vesical capillaries around the urinary bladder (*S. haematobium*). Hundreds of eggs are deposited daily. Eggs exit the host via the intestine with the feces (*S. mansoni*) or the urinary bladder, with the urine (*S. haematobium*) to continue the life cycle in compatible snails [12,20]. Numerous eggs are retained in the host tissue, inciting intense immune responses to the parasite egg antigens, characterized by granulomas formation around the eggs and progressive liver (*S. mansoni*) or urinary bladder (*S. haematobium*) tissue damage and fibrosis [21], and dominated by Th2 cytokines [14,15].

Skewing of the immune responses of patently infected hosts towards the Th2 axis may be the reason whereby infection with schistosomes increases the severity of subsequent infection with other pathogens namely *Plasmodium falciparum, Leishmania, Toxoplasma gondii, Mycobacteria, Entamoeba histolytica, Staphylococcus aureus,* or *Salmonella* [22, and references therein]. Schistosomiasis also may predispose individuals to infection with human immunodeficiency (HIV) and hepatitis C (HCV) virus, and increases resulting disease persistence and severity [2,23,24]. Individuals with schistosomiasis haematobium are at great risk for HIV infection, and for cancer development [24,25], afflictions all requiring robust Th1 responses for control and elimination [26].

2.2. Control

2.2.1. *Molluscicides*

Schistosome species require 2 hosts, a definitive mammalian and an intermediate freshwater snail host, for completion of the life cycle. *Schistosoma mansoni* and *S. haematobium* eggs release the miracidium, which must find a snail of the genus *Biomphalaria* and *Bulinus*, respectively for asexual reproduction, whereby infection of a compatible snail with a single miracidium results in production of thousands of infective cercariae [12,20]. The prevalence of schistosomiasis is linked to compatible snail distribution. Accordingly, breaking the dreadful cycle may well be accomplished via elimination of the obligatory intermediate snail host.

Snails of the *Biomphalaria* and *Bulinus* spp. live under water, and all molluscicidal measures must take into account vegetation, fish, ducks, and other animals habitat, as well as water quality for drinking and irrigation, rendering control of snails with chemicals, such as acrolein, copper sulfate, and niclosamide, a particularly costly approach [2,27].

2.2.2. *Sanitation and health education*

People acquire schistosomiasis while farming, fishing, bathing, washing, and performing recreational activities in the vicinity of water bodies contaminated with infected snails. Accordingly, safe water supply, improved sanitation, and health education are mandatory in order to effectively reduce (and eventually eliminate) the very significant global burden of disease due to schistosomiasis and other helminthic parasites, yet are unavailable in numerous countries due to poor economical, social, and political conditions [2-4].

2.2.3. *Praziquantel*

Praziquantel (PZQ), a pyrazino-isoquinoline derivative, FW 312.41, is practically now the single cost-affordable, and relatively safe and effective oral drug for mass treatment of hundreds of millions of individuals afflicted with schistosomiasis mansoni, schistosomiasis haematobium, and schistosomiasis japonicum as well [2-4,21]. Due to its hydrophobic nature and small size, PZQ inserts itself into the parasite outer lipid bilayer membrane, leading to its vacuolization, blebbing, and disruption [28]. Several reports documented the ability of PZQ to bind and polymerise actin [29-34]. Actin-based membrane skeleton (the fence) lies beneath the inner leaflet of the plasma membrane [35], and accordingly PZQ-parasite actin binding and subsequent polymerization may explain the severe muscle contraction and the paralysis worms undergo immediately upon exposure in vitro to PZQ. This mode of action, if proven to be true, suggests that PZQ treatment might not be entirely safe for children, persons with cardiovascular afflictions, and pregnant women [36].

Even if absolutely and entirely safe, PZQ treatment is not 100% proof and does not prevent reinfection or diminishes prevalence [37], necessitating periodic examination and repeated treatments, and thus, exacerbating the possiblity of the emergence of parasite resistance to the drug, a threat that has already materialized in several settings [38,39].

2.2.4. *Vaccine status – Documented target: The lung-stage schistosomula*

The hope for development of a schistosomiasis vaccine stems from the strong, and reproducible, protective immunity obtained after immunization of experimental hosts with radiation-attenuated (RA) cercariae [1,40], and the documented human resistance to infection (endemic normals), or reinfection after chemotherapy [41-43]. Sera and spleen cells of RA-vaccinated, and worm antigens-protectively immunized mice were used for identification of the potential protective target antigens. These studies resulted in identification, cloning, gene expression and assessment of protective potential of a plethora of molecules, among which *S. mansoni* irradiation associated vaccine antigen, IrV-5 [44], glutathione-S-transferase, GST [45], triose phosphate isomerase, TPI [46,47], paramyosin [48], fatty acid binding protein, Sm 14 [49], the surface membrane antigen Sm23 [50], the calcium-dependent cysteine protease, calpain [51], enolase [52,53], and calreticulin [54-56]. Reactivity of serum antibodies and peripheral blood mononuclear cells of resistant humans with fractionated worm molecules succeeded in identification of *S. mansoni* glyceraldehyde 3-phosphate dehydrogenase [57-61] as a potential candidate vaccine antigen. These molecules were used in conjunction with different adjuvants, namely complete (CFA) and incomplete (IFA) Freund's adjuvant for mouse immunization, leading to only hardly significant ($P < 0.05$) of some 30-35% reduction of challenge worm burden. Except for Sm23, these molecules are all cytosolic, and the poor protective capacity was ascribed to their inability to interact with the host immune system effector molecules.

Sm 23, an outer *S. mansoni* surface membrane antigen was among the molecules thought to be a target of protective immunity and of potential importance due to its residence at the host-parasite interface [50]. The full length molecule in a plasmid or recombinant form failed to lead to highly significant, consistent, or reproducible protection despite of their use in combination with a number of different adjuvants [62-64]. The *S. mansoni* integral surface membrane proteins tetraspanins (TSP)-1 and TSP-2 encoding cDNA were cloned, sequenced, and expressed and shown to elicit protection levels of 57% and 64% (TSP-2) and 34% and 52% (TSP-1) for mean adult worm burdens and liver egg burdens, respectively, over two independent trials in CBA/CaH mice [65]. The protection levels were not reproduced using *S. japonicum* counterpart, whereby mice immunized with the recombinant protein of a single TSP-2 subclass showed no protection, while immunization with a mixture of seven recombinant TSP-2 subclasses provided a moderate protection [66]. A recent study used *S. mansoni* TSP-2 extracellular loop 2 region in conjunction with alum and CpG as adjuvants leading to extremely variable protection levels against challenge infection within cohorts of highly inbred C57BL/6 mice [67]. An *S. mansoni* stomatin-like protein, a tegument protein located at the host-parasite interface, engendered in immunized mice a partial protection of 30-32%, associated with specific IgG1 and IgG2a antibodies and elevated production of IFN-g and tumor necrosis factor (TNF), while no IL-4 production was detected, suggesting a Th1-predominant immune response [68]. A schistosomular tegument preparation (Smteg) was used for C57BL/6 mice immunization, subcutaneously, on days 0, 15, and 30, resulting in significant antibody production, increased percentage of CD4 + IFN-g+ and CD4 + IL-10+ cells in spleen and increased production of IFN-g and IL-10 by spleen cells, but failed to reduce parasite burden, female fecundity and morbidity [69].

Sm23-, tetraspanins-, and other tegument-associated molecules- based protection was ascribed to specific antibody interaction with the molecules residing at the host-parasite interface, followed by binding to effector cells, which are able to elicit vigorous complement, and antibody-dependent cell-mediated cytotoxicity (ADCC) [65,67]. Indeed, ADCC was shown to be effective in killing a substantial proportion of 3-, 18- and sometimes 24-hr-old schistosomula [70-76], a phenomenon of limited in vivo relevance since larvae of that age still reside in the epidermis, impervious to any immune attack. On the other hand, older larvae, migrating schistosomula, pre-adut and adult worms surface membrane antigens are inaccessible to antibody binding [77,78], and thus, not threatened by ADCC. According, surface membrane, like cytosolic, antigens may not be considered for effective vaccination against schistosome infection.

No vaccine antigens appeared available, while we were striken by the paradox of lung-stage schistosomula being documented as the target of innate and RA vaccine immunity [1,40], and obtaining nutrients essentially via the tegument, while their surface membrane are entirely hidden, inaccessible to specific antibody binding.

3. The enigma of the lung-stage schistosomula

3.1. Lung-stage schistosomula strive without feeding in lung capillaries while surface membrane molecules are entirely hidden, inaccessible to specific antibody binding

Migrating schistosomula usually do not ingest erythrocytes because of their undersized mouth [79], and import sugar, fatty acids, and other nutrients directly across their tegument and into their internal tissues via membrane-spanning transporters [80-82]. Paradoxically, no specific antibody is able to bind to lung-stage larvae surface membrane antigens, as judged by several serological tests, namely indirect membrane immunofluorescence [1,40,77,78,83-89]. We were unable to visualize the presence of the glucose transporter

SGTP4 on the surface membrane of intact in vitro cultured or ex vivo 5 -7 day-old schistosomula, using specific antibodies and indirect membrane immunofluorescence [90]. Entire failure of larval surface membrane antigen detection does not give support to the contention that the tegument is bounded externally by a single lipid bilayer, overlain by a laminate secretion containing numerous proteins and molecular complexes [82,91], and was previously ascribed to shedding of antigenic molecules [86], masking by host proteins [85,88], or intrinsic biochemical modifications of the outer membrane [77,83,84,87, 89].

3.2. Attempts to expose the lung-stage and adult worm surface membrane antigens to specific antibody binding

In an attempt to overcome the lack of exposure of *S. mansoni* and *S. haematobium* lung stage larvae apical membrane antigens to specific antibody binding, we started by manipulating potential cues for increased surface antigenic expression, such as lack of glucose and amino acids, and extremes of pH or HCO_3^- concentration. All such trials failed to alter the negligible *S. mansoni* larval reactivity with RA vaccine and infection sera in membrane indirect immunofluorescence (IF). It was then thought that incubation of ex-vivo lung stage schistosomula in strongly hydrophobic medium might induce exposure of outer surface membrane hydrophobic sites, where antigenic molecules could be sequestered. Lung-stage schistosomula were, therefore, incubated with sera diluted in sterile corn oil. It is of note that corn oil essentially consists of poly- (linoleic acid, 45.9 to 55.5 %), and mono- (olecic acid, 28.4 to 36.9 %) unsaturated fatty acids, and contains 1 to 2% unsaponifiables particularly rich in sterols and tocopherols. *Schistosoma mansoni* [92] and *S. haematobium* (Figure 1) ex-vivo lung-stage schistosomula could readily bind specific antibodies of RA vaccine or infection sera in the fluorescent antibody test, following incubation in corn-oil in a concentration- and time-dependent manner.

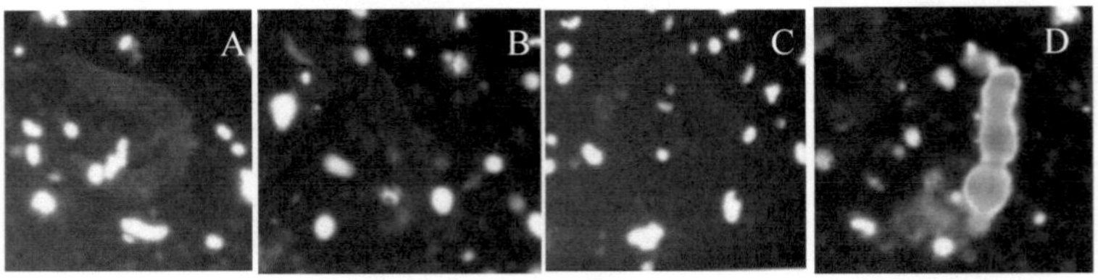

Figure 1. Assessment of the serological reactivity of *S. haematobium* lung-stage schistosomula by IF. Seven days ex vivo larvae incubated with control (A,C) or RA vaccine (B,D) serum diluted 1:50 in RPMI medium, before (A,B) or following incubation for 6 hr with 90% oil (C,D) were tested in IF and photographed under ultraviolet microscopy. x 200.

Since incubation of lung-stage parasites in corn oil led to exposure of antigenic sites in a concentration and time-dependent fashion, it was suggested that corn oil lipids may mediate efflux of cholesterol or phospholipids from the worm outer membrane, leading to changes in lateral diffusion of surface antigens that resulted into a dramatic increase in the avidity of antibody binding. Treatment with the membrane-impermeable, cholesterol-extracting drug methyl-b-cyclodextrin (MBCD), followed by visualization of surface membrane cholesterol by staining with filipin III, a fluorescent polyene antibiotic, widely used for the detection and the quantitation of cholesterol in biomembranes, allowed us to examine the role of cholesterol in surface membrane antigen sequestration of *S. mansoni* and *S. haematobium* ex vivo lung-stage larvae. Evaluation of cholesterol content and distribution by filipin staining demonstrated that MBCD efficiently extracts cholesterol from the surface membrane of *S. mansoni* and *S. haematobium* lung-stage larvae [93,94]. Treatment of *S. mansoni* ex-vivo lung-stage larvae with MBCD consistently and reproducibly led to considerable binding of specific antibodies to the outer membrane surface. The data, thus, suggest that depletion of cholesterol from the outer membrane of *S. mansoni* lung-stage schistosomula corrects their failure to bind antibodies in the fluorescent antibody test. However, *S. haematobium* larvae treated with 2.5, 5.0, or 10 mM MBCD were consistently negative following incubation with either control or RA serum in the fluorescent antibody test. Hence, the results indicated that almost complete depletion of cholesterol from the surface membrane of *S. haematobium* larvae did not modify the negligible binding of specific antibodies by the surface membrane antigens. This means that *S. haematobium* and *S. mansoni* ex vivo lung-stage larvae differ regarding the contribution of cholesterol to the sequestration of surface membrane antigens [93,94].

3.3. Solving the schistosomula lung-stage enigma and predicting the existence of a parasite tegument-associated neutral sphingomyelinase (nSMase)

The data together strongly supported the contention that antigenic molecules persist on the surface of ex-vivo lung-stage schistosomula [89-91], yet are entirely inaccessible to specific antibody binding, in part due to cholesterol sequestration. Surface membrane antigens of *S. mansoni* and *S. haematobium* ex vivo lung schistosomula were, however, readily exposed to specific antibody binding following incubation in corn oil as mentioned above. It was hypothesized that corn oil unsaturated fatty acids (FA) might activate parasite surface membrane-bound neutral sphingomyelinase (nSMase), leading to hydrolysis of surface membrane sphingomyelin (SM), and subsequent decrease in outer bilayer lipid rigidity and permeability. At variance from MBCD, incubation of lung-stage schistosomula with unsaturated FA, such as corn and olive oil, or arachidonic acid (ARA), led to exposure of the, otherwise concealed, surface membrane antigens of *S. mansoni* and *S. haematobium* alike. In that respect, *S. haematobium* appeared more sensitive than *S. mansoni*, requiring lower unsaturated FA concentrations and shorter incubation periods [95, and references therein].

Evaluation of cholesterol amount and distribution by the filipin staining method indicated that unsaturated FA did not appear to elicit exposure of schistosomular surface membrane antigens via cholesterol extraction, as previously suggested. While a definite proof needs and remains to be established, some lines of evidence support the hypothesis that unsaturated FA might elicit larval surface membrane antigen exposure via their ability to stimulate a putative tegument-associated nSMase, with subsequent SM hydrolysis, and access of antibodies [95,96].

We have been able to demonstrate that 1- intact healthy ex vivo schistosomula, displaying equilibrium in SM synthesis and hydrolysis, allow molecules of less than 600 Da to access their surface membrane molecules. 2- Ex vivo larvae exposed to conditions conducive to nSMase inactivation (pH less than 7.2, high concentrations of nitric oxide or hydrogen peroxide), do not allow neither antibodies nor even very small molecules (less than 600 Da) to access their surface membrane molecules [96]. Sphingomyelin appears critical in maintaining the rigidity and impermeability of the parasite outer lipid bilayer, likely via the ability of hydroxyl and amide groups in the interfacial region of sphingolipids to form with water molecules a tight netwok of hydrogen bonds [96, and references therein]. Recently, quasi-elastic and inelastic neutron scattering experiments on *S. mansoni* and *S. haematobium* worms and larvae have been performed. The obtained experimental findings suggest that the larva-medium interaction is triggered by the hydrogen bond network. Furthermore, the strength of that hydrogen bond network-based interaction appeared to be higher for *S. mansoni* larvae than adult worms and for *S. mansoni* than *S. haematobium* [Federica Migliardo, Unpublished Observations]. 3- Inhibition of ex vivo larvae SM synthesis or moderate nSMase activation (exposure to low concentrations of unsaturated FA, especially ARA) allows specific antibody access and visualization of surface membrane antigens. Exposure of ex vivo larvae to conditions conducive to excessive nSMase activation (hypoxia, high concentrations of unsaturated FA, notably ARA) lead to their irreversible attrition [96, and references therein].

3.4. Evidence for the existence of parasite tegument-associated nSMase and its activation by arachidonic acid

In 2006, we predicted, and provided evidence for, the existence of a schistosome tegument-associated Mg^{2+}-dependent nSMase, which is able to hydrolyze some SM molecules, thus allowing nutrients, but not host antibodies, to access proteins at the host-parasite interface [96]. Excessive activation of the elusive nSMase using the unsaturated FA, ARA led to larval and adult worm surface membrane antigens exposure and eventual attrition [95-97]. The identification and sequence of *S. mansoni* putative nSMase was reported by Berriman et al. in 2009 [98; Accession number XP_002578732.1]. The molecule of 70.99 kDa was shown to consist of 631 amino acids (aa) with an N-terminal, 300 aa Mg^{++}-dependent exonuclease/endonuclease/ phosphatase (EEP) superfamily catalytic domain, and predicted 7 transmembrane regions at aa locations 355-377, 392-414, 435-457, 461-483, 527-549, 564-586 and 595-617 (genedb. org/ gene/ Smp_162880). The *S. mansoni* putative nSMase showed about 52% homology with the amino terminal 300 aa of *Mus musculus* and human nSMase 1, which consists of 419 and 423 aa, respectively, an exonuclease/endonuclease/phosphatase superfamily domain at the N-terminus, and two transmembrane domains at the C-terminus.

Using primers based on the published sequence of *S. mansoni* nSMase, El Halbousy, Tallima, and El Ridi (personal communication) succeeded in cloning and sequencing 836 bp near the 5′ end of *S. haematobium* nSMase-encoding mRNA. The predicted aa sequences corresponded to aa18- aa277 in the *S. mansoni* counterpart with 96% identities and 98% positives (Figure 2), and contained the conserved domains characterizing the EEP superfamily.

http://dx.doi.org/10.5772/52922

```
SHnSM 1    FPSSTVRKEDRVNAIAAXLSVGDFDVILLQEIWLESDYRKLRNILDEKYPYSNYFYCNLI 60
           FPSSTVRKEDRVNAIA+  LSVGDFDVILLQEIWLESDYRKLRNILDEKYPYSNYFYCNLI
SMnSM 18   FPSSTVRKEDRVNAIASKLSVGDFDVILLQEIWLESDYRKLRNILDEKYPYSNYFYCNLI 77

SHnSM 61   GTGMCIFSKWTIECVFTHPFTTNGYPHLIHQADYYCGKGIGLARITSKEGFRINFYVTHL 120
           GTGMCIFSKWTIECVFTHPFT NGYPHLIHQADYYCGKGIGLARITSKEGFRINFYVTHL
SMnSM 78   GTGMCIFSKWTIECVFTHPFTANGYPHLIHQADYYCGKGIGLARITSKEGFRINFYVTHL 137

SHnSM 121  IARYELDRMLDKYNGHRISQLVEIMEFVRMTSTGSDAIIITGDFNLESNTSAIELFSTSL 180
           IARYELDRMLD+YNGHRISQLVE+MEFVRMTSTGSDAIIITGDFNLESNTSAIELFSTSL
SMnSM 138  IARYELDRMLDRYNGHRISQLVEVMEFVRMTSTGSDAIIITGDFNLESNTSAIELFSTSL 197

SHnSM 181  KLSDAWLNNTVALKNTNITELESEGCTCDRADNPYRNQLWTNTYGNGERLDYIFYRSGPS 240
           KLSDAWLNNTVALKNTNIT+LESEGCTCDRADNPYRNQLWTNTYGNGERLDYIFYRSGPS
SMnSM 198  KLSDAWLNNTVALKNTNITDLESEGCTCDRADNPYRNQLWTNTYGNGERLDYIFYRSGPS 257

SHnSM 241  IIDSFHIPSYAKLVCDSCWF 260
           IIDSF+IPSYAKLVC+SCW
Sbjct 258  IIDSFYIPSYAKLVCNSCWL 277
```

Figure 2. Homology between predicted amino acid sequences of *S. mansoni* (SMnSM) and *S. haematobium* (SHnSM) neutral sphingomyelinase.

A systematically improved high quality genome and transcriptome of the human blood fluke *S. mansoni* was recently reported by Protasio et al. (unpublished observations), whereby sequence for *S. mansoni* putative nSMase was now shown to encode 431 (CCD60196.1) and not 631 (XP_002578732.1) aa and 100% identity with the latter sequence only for the first 345 aa, as only 2 transmembrane domains were identified near the carboxyl end, between aa 325 and 375.

It is of note that the whole-genome sequence of *S. haematobium* was recently published [99], and reported the coding sequence (1038 bp) of an *S. haematobium* putative neutral sphingomyelinase (http://www.schistodb.net; Sha_103241), encoding 345 aa, with 3 transmembrane domains at the carboxyl end. Blasting of our SHnSM sequences with Sha_103241 revealed 94-97% homology. However, the sretch of SHnSm aa33-116 (highlighted in Figure 2), which contained EEP superfamily signature sites and showed complete homology with the *S. mansoni* counterpart, was lacking in Sha_103241 published sequence.

Antibodies specific to *S. mansoni* nSMase were generated in mice, immunized with peptides based on the molecule predicted aa sequence, synthesized as multiple antigen peptide (MAP) constructs. We were able to confirm the presence of the enzyme in adult male and female *S. mansoni* and *S. haematobium* tegument as judged by enzyme-linked immunosorbent assay (ELISA) and membrane and cytoplasmic IF. We were also the first to measure nSMase enzymatic activity in Triton X-100-solubilized surface membrane (Sup 1) and whole worm soluble (SWAP) molecules of male and female *S. mansoni* and *S. haematobium*. Neutral, but no acidic, sphingomyelinase activity was readily detectable by the Amplex Red Sphingomyelinase Assay, and increased with incubation time and protein amount. The nSMase activity of Sup 1 and SWAP of male and female *S. mansoni* and *S. haematobium* adult worms was significantly ($P < 0.05 - < 0.0001$) increased following exposure to 125 or 250 mM linoleic acid, ARA, docosahexaenoic acid, or phosphatidyl serine, with ARA consistently showing the highest nSMase activating potential [100].

4. Arachidonic acid as a remedy for schistosomiasis

Since incubation of *S. mansoni* and *S. haematobium* ex vivo larvae [95,96] and adult worms [97] with ARA leads to exposure of surface membrane antigens and eventual attrition, it was rational to propose ARA for chemotherapy of schistosomiasis. ARA could be schistosomicidal per se, and additionally would expose the parasite surface membrane molecules to host antibodies-mediated attack, thus eliciting drug and immune system synergy.

In our studies, pure ARA from Sigma was used for in vitro and preliminary in vivo studies, while ARA from Martek was used for in vivo studies [101,102]. We have demonstrated that 5 mM pure ARA (Sigma) leads to irreversible killing of ex vivo larval, juvenile, pre-adult and adult *S. mansoni* and *S. haematobium* worms, within 1- 5 hr, depending on the parasite age, and the fetal calf serum concentration. ARA-mediated worm attrition was prevented by nSMase inhibitors such as $CaCl_2$ and GW4869. Electron microscopy studies revealed entire disruption of the outer lipid bilayers, the strength of which correlated with ARA concentration. These consistent and reproducible findings indicate that ARA is schistosomicidal per se [101].

ARA-mediated *S. mansoni* and *S. haematobium* worm in vitro attrition was reproduced in vivo whereby a series of 20 independent experiments, using BALB/c or C57BL/6 mice or Syrian hamsters, indicated that oral administration of 300-2500 mg/kg ARA in a pure form (Sigma), included in infant formula (Nestle), or capsules (X Factor, Molecular Nutrition), on 2 consecutive days, consistently led to between 50 and 80% decrease in *S. mansoni* or *S. haematobium* worm burden [101,102]. ARA-mediated attrition in vivo appeared to be associated with high titers of serum antibodies to tegumental antigens, because it was significantly higher when treatment was started at 8, rather than 5 or 6, week post infection with *S. mansoni*. Immune responses to adult worm tegumental antigens are certainly powerful in adults and children with patent or chronic schistosomiasis, and ARA is already marketed for human use in USA and Canada for proper development of newborns, and muscle growth of athletes. Accordingly, it is recommended to start pre-clinical and clinical studies in human volunteers for development of ARA as a safe and cost-effective remedy to schistosomiasis, especially that no ARA-related adverse effects were seen in any experiment in mice or hamsters [101-103].

5. Larval excretory-secretory products as vaccine candidates

Schistosome cytosolic and surface membrane antigens are entirely hidden, inaccessible to the host immune system effectors. As spelled out by Patrick Skelly [104], "schistosomes have achieved invisibility", and if it were not for the parasite "scent", the excretory-secretory products (ESP), a schistosomiasis vaccine would be as good as over.

Excretory-secretory products of cercariae, in vitro cultured and ex vivo lung-stage schistosomula, and adult worms of *S. mansoni, S. japonicum* [8,17,105-111], and *S. haematobium* as well [99] have been identified in several studies, and were found to be dominated by actin, enolase, aldolase, GST,TPI, glyceraldehyde-3 phosphate dehydrogenase (SG3PDH), thioredoxin peroxidease (TPX) = peroxyredoxin, proteases, and calcium-binding proteins, namely calpain.

Cercarial ESP would activate innate immune cells in the epidermis and dermis [8-11,111-117], but would not be targeted by antibody or complement products in the blood- and lymph-free epidermis. In the dermis, larval ESP may interact with host innate effectors, such as natural antibodies, serum lectins and complement components, resulting into inflammation that would facilitate the parasite entry into dermal blood capillaries. Schistosomula then migrate via the venous system in relatively large vessels, whereby ESP are quickly "washed" away by neutrophils and monocytes. In contrast, lung-stage larvae ESP likely stagnate in the narrow, convoluted, and notably thin-walled lung capillaries and liver sinusoids. These sites are the most strenuous of the journey, an occasion for the parasite to get rid of the less fit "members", and an explanation for the lung-stage and pre-adult larvae being documented as the target of innate and acquired resistance to schistosomiasis [1,118]. Adult worms reside in vessels, which are neither narrow nor thin-walled, and accordingly, the large ESP amounts they release are rapidly pinocytosed or phagocytosed, and transported away from the worms for stimulation of rather innocuous immune responses in the spleen, the principal target for intravascular antigens.

6. The plausible mechanism of innate and immune attrition of invading larvae

Migrating larvae ESP presented by blood monocytes and dendritic cells trigger Th lymphocytes in host spleen for production of predominantly Th1 (IFN-g and TNF) and Th17 (IL-17) cytokines [14,15,17-19], especially if the host was previously RA-vaccinated [16,118] or immunized with vaccine candidate antigens in conjunction with Th1 adjuvants [62-68]. Additionally, larval ESP- antibody complexes may activate immune effector cells via FcR binding. Stimulated monocytes produce nitric oxide and reactive oxygen products [119], which are lethal to near-by schistosomules; however, these toxic molecules inhibit the parasite tegument-associated nSMase activity, leading to outer membrane entire impermeability [95,96,120,121]. Neutrophils recruited and activated by Th17 cytokines likely ensnare larvae in their extracellular traps, yet secrete proteases and other enzymes that might all be ineffective because of the worm tight lipid bilayer and inaccessibility of surface membrane molecules [119,122,123].

Eosinophils also produce extracellular traps, and their basic molecules would be severely toxic to captured schistomula [124,125]. Basophils release cytotoxic basic molecules, and most importantly, pharmacologic mediators able to modulate endothelial integrity, thus encouraging larvae to escape extravascularly to a certain demise [126]. Indeed, that attrition mechanism was shown to be of great importance in resistance to challenge infection in the RA model [118]. However, eosinophils and basophils are recruited and activated by type 2 cytokines [125,126], and thus, are prevented from active participation in the hunt for developing larvae [1,19] following infection of naive and antigens/Th1 adjuvant-immunized mice. Nevertheless, attempts to vaccinate mice against schistosomiasis uniformly aim at enhancing Th1 immune responses, in spite of the documented role of Th2 cytokines, namely IL-4, in protection of RA immunized mice [127-130]. Also in rats, sterile resistance to *S. mansoni* is associated with production of IL-4, IL-5, and IL-13, while susceptibility is accompanied with elevated expression of IFN-g [131,132]. In humans, a good association was previously observed between serum IgE production and resistance to infection after chemotherapy [41-43]. Indeed, Fallon et al. [133] reported that "adult resistance and child susceptibly to reinfection after chemotherapy have been described for all 3 *Schistosoma* species that most commonly infect man. For all 3 parasite species, the immunological correlates of this age-dependent resistance are associated with type 2 responses". These findings were entirely confirmed in recent studies [134-136].

7. The road to a sterilizing schistosomiasis vaccine

Larval ESP are innumerable, among which we have selected those eliciting the weakest Th1 and Th17 responses, namely SG3PDH in a recombinant (rSG3PDH) form and a TPX MAP construct [19,110]. Nevetheless, it was critical to use an adjuvant that would skew the larval immune responses towards the Th2 axis. In contrast to incomplete Freund's adjuvant, alum, polyinosinic-polycytidylic acid, and peptidoglycan, the Th2 master cytokine, thymic stromal lymphopoietin (TSLP), succeeded in directing the ESP-mediated immune responses towards a Th2-biased profile in prototypical Th1 (C57BL/6) and Th2 (BALB/c) mice [110,137]. Thereafter, we have immunized outbred, akin to humans, mice with rSG3PDH and TPX MAP in conjunction with the type 2 cytokines, TSLP, IL-25, or IL-33 [138, and references therein]. Results of 8 independent experiments indicated that these formulations elicited IgM, IgG1, and IgA specific antibodies, and an increase in ex vivo spleen cells release of IL-4, IL-5, and IL-13 correlated with consistent, reproducible, and highly significant ($P < 0.0001$) reduction of 62% to 78% in challenge *S. mansoni* worm burden [138]. Similar studies using *S. haematobium* are now in progress.

8. Conclusion

Improved selection of larval ESP, singly or in a mixture, and type 2 adjuvant is expected to result into a sterilizing vaccine against schistosome infection. Concurrent development of ARA, a nutrient, a component of our cell membranes, for chemotherapy of infection in un-

http://dx.doi.org/10.5772/52922

immunized individuals, will likely lead to full control, and eventual elimination of schistosomiasis.

Experiments. related to novel approaches to therapy and vaccination were supported, in part, by the Science and Technology Development Fund, Egypt, grants No. 144 and 2073 to R. El Ridi. We are indebted to Mr. Abdel Badih Foda for help and assistance.

Author details

Rashika El Ridi and Hatem Tallima

*Address all correspondence to: rashikaelridi@hotmail.com, rashika@mailer.eun.eg

Zoology Department, Faculty of Science, Cairo University, Cairo, Egypt

References

[1] von Lichtenberg F, Sher A, McIntyre S. A lung model of schistosome immunity in mice. American Journal of Pathology 1977;87(1): 105-123.

[2] King CH. Parasites and poverty: the case of schistosomiasis. Acta Tropica 2010;113(2): 95-104.

[3] Hotez P. Enlarging the "Audacious Goal": elimination of the world's high prevalence neglected tropical diseases. Vaccine 2011;29 Suppl 4:D104-110.

[4] Gray DJ, McManus DP, Li Y, Williams GM, Bergquist R, Ross AG. Schistosomiasis elimination: lessons from the past guide the future. Lancet Infectious Diseases 2010;10(10):733-736.

[5] He YX, Chen L, Ramaswamy K. Schistosoma mansoni, S. haematobium, and S. japonicum: early events associated with penetration and migration of schistosomula through human skin. Experimental Parasitolology 2002;102(2): 99-108.

[6] Curwen RS, Wilson RA. Invasion of skin by schistosome cercariae: some neglected facts. Trends in Parasitolology 2003;19(2): 63-66.

[7] Stirewalt MA. Schistosoma mansoni: cercaria to schistosomule. Advances in Parasitology 1974;12: 115-182.

[8] Harrop R, Jennings N, Mountford AP, Coulson PS, Wilson RA. Characterization, cloning and immunogenicity of antigens released by transforming cercariae of Schistosoma mansoni. Parasitology 2000;121 (Pt 4): 385-394.

[9] Pivarcsi A, Kemény L, Dobozy A. Innate immune functions of the keratinocytes. A review. Acta Microbiologica Immunologica Hungarica 2004;51(3): 303-310.

[10] Chen L, Rao KV, He YX, Ramaswamy K. Skin-stage schistosomula of Schistosoma mansoni produce an apoptosis-inducing factor that can cause apoptosis of T cells. Journal of Biological Chemistry 2002;277(37): 34329-34335.

[11] Paveley RA, Aynsley SA, Cook PC, Turner JD, Mountford AP. Fluorescent imaging of antigen released by a skin-invading helminth reveals differential uptake and activation profiles by antigen presenting cells. PLoS Neglected Tropical Diseases 2009;3(10): e528.

[12] Schistosoma, blood fluke. http://www.metapathogen.com/schistosoma/ (accessed 22 April 2012).

[13] Rheinberg CE, Moné H, Caffrey CR, Imbert-Establet D, Jourdane J, Ruppel A. Schistosoma haematobium, S. intercalatum, S. japonicum, S. mansoni, and S. rodhaini in mice: relationship between patterns of lung migration by schistosomula and perfusion recovery of adult worms. Parasitology Research 1998;84(4): 338-342.

[14] Grzych JM, Pearce E, Cheever A, Caulada ZA, Caspar P, Heiny S, Lewis F, Sher A. Egg deposition is the major stimulus for the production of Th2 cytokines in murine schistosomiasis mansoni. Journal of Immunology 1991;146(4): 1322-1327.

[15] Pearce EJ, Caspar P, Grzych JM, Lewis FA, Sher A. Downregulation of Th1 cytokine production accompanies induction of Th2 responses by a parasitic helminth, Schistosoma mansoni. Journal of Experimental Medicine 1991;173(1): 159-166.

[16] Mountford AP, Harrop R, Wilson RA. Antigens derived from lung-stage larvae of Schistosoma mansoni are efficient stimulators of proliferation and gamma interferon secretion by lymphocytes from mice vaccinated with attenuated larvae. Infection and Immunity 1995;63(5): 1980-1986.

[17] Harrop R, Coulson PS, Wilson RA. Characterization, cloning and immunogenicity of antigens released by lung-stage larvae of Schistosoma mansoni. Parasitology1999;118 (Pt 6): 583-594.

[18] Tallima H, Salah M, Guirguis FR, El Ridi R. Transforming growth factor-beta and Th17 responses in resistance to primary murine schistosomiasis mansoni. Cytokine 2009;48(3): 239-245.

[19] El Ridi R, Tallima H, Mahana N, Dalton JP. Innate immunogenicity and in vitro protective potential of Schistosoma mansoni lung schistosomula excretory-secretory candidate vaccine antigens. Microbes and Infection 2010;12(10): 700-709.

[20] Walker AJ. Insights into the functional biology of schistosomes. Parasites and Vectors 2011;4: 203.

[21] Andersson KL, Chung RT. Hepatic schistosomiasis. Current Treatment Options in Gastroenterology 2007;10: 504-512.

[22] Abruzzi A, Fried B. Coinfection of Schistosoma (Trematoda) with bacteria, protozoa and helminths. Advances in Parasitology 2011;77: 1-85.

[23] Farid A, Al-Sherbiny M, Osman A, Mohamed N, Saad A, Shata MT, Lee DH, Prince AM, Strickland GT. Schistosoma infection inhibits cellular immune responses to core HCV peptides. Parasite Immunology 2005;27(5): 189-196.

[24] Secor WE. The effects of schistosomiasis on HIV/AIDS infection, progression and transmission. Current Opinion in HIV and AIDS 2012;7(3): 254-259.

[25] Botelho MC, Machado JC, da Costa JM. Schistosoma haematobium and bladder cancer: what lies beneath? Virulence 2010;1(2): 84-87.

[26] El Ridi R, El Garem AA. Is an anti-Schistosoma haematobium vaccine necessary? International Journal for Parasitology 1999;29(4): 651-653.

[27] Davie J. Medical Ecology-Schistosomiasis. In Parasitic Diseases 5th Edition. Chapter 35. www.medicalecology.org/water/w_schist.htm

[28] Mehlhorn H, Becker B, Andrews P, Thomas H, Frenkel JK. In vivo and in vitro experiments on the effects of praziquantel on Schistosoma mansoni. A light and electron microscopic study. Arzneimittelforschung 1981;31(3a): 544-554.

[29] Linder E, Thors C. Schistosoma mansoni: praziquantel-induced tegumental lesion exposes actin of surface spines and allows binding of actin depolymerizing factor, gelsolin. Parasitology 1992; 105(Pt 1): 71-79.

[30] Tallima H, El Ridi R. Praziquantel binds Schistosoma mansoni adult worm actin. International Journal of Antimicrobial Agents 2007;29(5): 570-575.

[31] Tallima H, El Ridi R. Re: is actin the praziquantel receptor? International Journal of Antimicrobial Agents 2007;30(6): 566-567.

[32] Pica-Mattoccia L, Valle C, Basso A, Troiani AR, Vigorosi F, Liberti P, Festucci A, Cioli D. Cytochalasin D abolishes the schistosomicidal activity of praziquantel. Experimental Parasitology 2007;115(4): 344-351.

[33] Pica-Mattoccia L, Orsini T, Basso A, Festucci A, Liberti P, Guidi A, Marcatto-Maggi AL, Nobre-Santana S, Troiani AR, Cioli D, Valle C. Schistosoma mansoni: lack of correlation between praziquantel-induced intra-worm calcium influx and parasite death. Experimental Parasitology 2008;119(3): 332-335.

[34] Gnanasekar M, Salunkhe AM, Mallia AK, He YX, Kalyanasundaram R. Praziquantel affects the regulatory myosin light chain of Schistosoma mansoni. Antimicrobial Agents and Chemotherapy 2009;53(3): 1054-1060.

[35] Viola A, Gupta N. Tether and trap: regulation of membrane-raft dynamics by actin-binding proteins. Nature Reviews Immunology 2007;7(11): 889-896.

[36] Allen HE, Crompton DW, de Silva N, LoVerde PT, Olds GR. New policies for using anthelmintics in high risk groups. Trends in Parasitology 2002;18(9): 381-382.

[37] Landouré A, Dembélé R, Goita S, Kané M, Tuinsma M, Sacko M, Toubali E, French MD, Keita AD, Fenwick A, Traoré MS, Zhang Y. Significantly reduced intensity of infection but persistent prevalence of schistosomiasis in a highly endemic region in Mali after repeated treatment. PLoS Neglected Tropical Diseases 2012;6(7): e1774.

[38] Melman SD, Steinauer ML, Cunningham C, Kubatko LS, Mwangi IN, Wynn NB, Mutuku MW, Karanja DM, Colley DG, Black CL, Secor WE, Mkoji GM, Loker ES. Reduced susceptibility to praziquantel among naturally occurring Kenyan isolates of Schistosoma mansoni. PLoS Neglected Tropical Diseases 2009;3(8): e504.

[39] Pica-Mattoccia L, Doenhoff MJ, Valle C, Basso A, Troiani AR, Liberti P, Festucci A, Guidi A, Cioli D. Genetic analysis of decreased praziquantel sensitivity in a laboratory strain of Schistosoma mansoni. Acta Tropica 2009;111(1): 82-85.

[40] Wilson RA. The saga of schistosome migration and attrition. Parasitology 2009;136(12):1581-1592.

[41] Hagan P, Wilkins HA, Blumenthal UJ, Hayes RJ, Greenwood BM. Eosinophilia and resistance to Schistosoma haematobium in man. Parasite Immunology 1985;7(6): 625-632.

[42] Wilkins HA, Blumenthal UJ, Hagan P, Hayes RJ, Tulloch S. Resistance to reinfection after treatment of urinary schistosomiasis. Transactions of the Royal Society of Tropical Medicine and Hygiene 1987;81(1): 29-35.

[43] Kabatereine NB, Vennervald BJ, Ouma JH, Kemijumbi J, Butterworth AE, Dunne DW, Fulford AJ. Adult resistance to schistosomiasis mansoni: age-dependence of reinfection remains constant in communities with diverse exposure patterns. Parasitology1999;118 (Pt 1): 101-105.

[44] Soisson LM, Masterson CP, Tom TD, McNally MT, Lowell GH, Strand M. Induction of protective immunity in mice using a 62-kDa recombinant fragment of a Schistosoma mansoni surface antigen. Journal of Immunology 1992;149(11): 3612-3620.

[45] Balloul JM, Sondermeyer P, Dreyer D, Capron M, Grzych JM, Pierce RJ, Carvallo D, Lecocq JP, Capron A. Molecular cloning of a protective antigen of schistosomes. Nature 1987;326(6109): 149-153.

[46] Harn DA, Wei G, Oligino LD, Mitsuyama M, Gebremichael A, Richter D. A protective monoclonal antibody specifically recognizes and alters the catalytic activity of schistosome triose-phosphate isomerase. Journal of Immunology 1992;148(2): 562-567.

[47] Shoemaker C, Gross A, Gebremichael A, Harn D. cDNA cloning and functional expression of the Schistosoma mansoni protective antigen triose-phosphate isomerase. Proceedings of the National Academy of Sciences USA 1992;89(5): 1842-1846.

[48] Lanar DE, Pearce EJ, James SL, Sher A. Identification of paramyosin as schistosome antigen recognized by intradermally vaccinated mice. Science 1986;234(4776): 593-596.

[49] Moser D, Tendler M, Griffiths G, Klinkert MQ. A 14-kDa Schistosoma mansoni polypeptide is homologous to a gene family of fatty acid binding proteins. Journal of Biological Chemistry 1991;266(13):8447-8454.

[50] Reynolds SR, Shoemaker CB, Harn DA. T and B cell epitope mapping of Sm23, an integral membrane protein of Schistosoma mansoni. Journal of Immunology 1992;149(12) :3995-4001.

[51] Siddiqui AA, Zhou Y, Podesta RB, Karcz SR, Tognon CE, Strejan GH, Dekaban GA, Clarke MW. Characterization of Ca(2+)-dependent neutral protease (calpain) from human blood flukes, Schistosoma mansoni. Biochimica et Biophysica Acta 1993;1181(1): 37-44.

[52] El Ridi R, Abdel Tawab N, Guirguis N. Schistosoma mansoni: identification and protective immunity of adult worm antigens recognized by T lymphocytes of outbred Swiss mice immunized with irradiated cercariae. Experimental Parasitology 1993;76(3): 265-277.

[53] Abdel Tawab N. Identification and molecular characterization of protective antigens against murine schistosomiasis mansoni. PhD thesis. Faculty of Science, Cairo University;1994.

[54] Osman A, El Ridi R, Guirguis N, Dean DA. Identification of Schistosoma mansoni antigens recognized by T cells of C57BL/6 mice immunized with gamma-irradiated cercariae. Journal of Parasitology 1994;80 (3); 421-431.

[55] Osman A, El Ridi R, Guirguis N, Dean DA. Identification of Schistosoma mansoni antigens recognized by spleen cells of C57B1/6 mice immunized with ultraviolet-irradiated cercariae. International Journal for Parasitology 194;24(7): 943-950.

[56] El Gengehi N, El Ridi R, Tawab NA, El Demellawy M, Mangold BL. A Schistosoma mansoni 62-kDa band is identified as an irradiated vaccine T-cell antigen and characterized as calreticulin. Journal of Parasitology 2000;86(5): 993-1000.

[57] Dessein AJ, Begley M, Demeure C, Caillol D, Fueri J, dos Reis MG, Andrade ZA, Prata A, Bina JC. Human resistance to Schistosoma mansoni is associated with IgG reactivity to a 37-kDa larval surface antigen. Journal of Immunology 1988;140(8): 2727-2736.

[58] Goudot-Crozel V, Caillol D, Djabali M, Dessein AJ. The major parasite surface antigen associated with human resistance to schistosomiasis is a 37-kD glyceraldehyde-3P-dehydrogenase. Journal of Experimental Medicine 1989;170(6): 2065-2080.

[59] Charrier-Ferrara S, Caillol D, Goudot-Crozel V. Complete sequence of the Schistosoma mansoni glyceraldehyde-3-phosphate dehydrogenase gene encoding a major surface antigen. Molecular and Biochemical Parasitology 1992;56(2): 339-343.

[60] El Ridi R, Farouk F, Sherif M, Al-Sherbiny M, Osman A, El Gengehi N, Shoemaker CB. T and B cell reactivity to a 42-kDa protein is associated with human resistance to

both schistosomiasis mansoni and haematobium. Journal of Infectious Diseases 1998;177(5): 1364-1372.

[61] El Ridi R, Shoemaker CB, Farouk F, El Sherif NH, Afifi A. Human T- and B-cell responses to Schistosoma mansoni recombinant glyceraldehyde 3-phosphate dehydrogenase correlate with resistance to reinfection with S. mansoni or Schistosoma haematobium after chemotherapy. Infection and Immunity 2001;69(1): 237-244.

[62] Da'dara AA, Skelly PJ, Wang MM, Harn DA. Immunization with plasmid DNA encoding the integral membrane protein, Sm23, elicits a protective immune response against schistosome infection in mice. Vaccine 2001;20(3-4): 359-369.

[63] Da'dara AA, Skelly PJ, Fatakdawala M, Visovatti S, Eriksson E, Harn DA. Comparative efficacy of the Schistosoma mansoni nucleic acid vaccine, Sm23, following microseeding or gene gun delivery. Parasite Immunology 2002;24(4): 179-187.

[64] Da'Dara AA, Skelly PJ, Walker CM, Harn DA. A DNA-prime/protein-boost vaccination regimen enhances Th2 immune responses but not protection following Schistosoma mansoni infection. Parasite Immunology 2003;25(8-9): 429-437.

[65] Tran MH, Pearson MS, Bethony JM, Smyth DJ, Jones MK, Duke M, Don TA, McManus DP, Correa-Oliveira R, Loukas A. Tetraspanins on the surface of Schistosoma mansoni are protective antigens against schistosomiasis. Nature Medicine 2006;12(7): 835-840.

[66] Zhang W, Li J, Duke M, Jones MK, Kuang L, Zhang J, Blair D, Li Y, McManus DP. Inconsistent protective efficacy and marked polymorphism limits the value of Schistosoma japonicum tetraspanin-2 as a vaccine target. PLoS Neglegted Tropical Diseases 2011;5(5): e1166.

[67] Pearson MS, Pickering DA, McSorley HJ, Bethony JM, Tribolet L, Dougall AM, Hotez PJ, Loukas A. Enhanced protective efficacy of a chimeric form of the schistosomiasis vaccine antigen Sm-TSP-2. PLoS Neglegted Tropical Diseases 2012;6(3): e1564.

[68] Farias LP, Cardoso FC, Miyasato PA, Montoya BO, Tararam CA, Roffato HK, Kawano T, Gazzinelli A, Correa-Oliveira R, Coulson PS, Wilson RA, Oliveira SC, Leite LC. Schistosoma mansoni Stomatin like protein-2 is located in the tegument and induces partial protection against challenge infection. PLoS Neglected Tropical Diseases 2010;4(2): e597.

[69] Araujo JM, Melo TT, Sena IC, Alves CC, Araujo N, Durães FD, Oliveira SC, Fonseca CT. Schistosoma mansoni schistosomula tegument (Smteg) immunization in absence of adjuvant induce IL-10 production by CD4+ cells and failed to protect mice against challenge infection. Acta Tropica 2012; 124(2): 140-146. (PMID: 22842304).

[70] Butterworth AE, David JR, Franks D, Mahmoud AA, David PH, Sturrock RF, Houba V. Antibody-dependent eosinophil-mediated damage to 51Cr-labeled schistosomula of Schistosoma mansoni: damage by purified eosinophils. Journal of Experimental Medicine 1977;145(1): 136-150.

[71] Kassis AI, Aikawa M, Mahmoud AF. Mouse antibody-dependent eosinophil and macrophage adherence and damage to schistosomula of Schistosoma mansoni. Journal of Immunology 1979; 122(2): 398-405.

[72] Balloul JM, Pierce RJ, Grzych JM, Capron A. In vitro synthesis of a 28 kilodalton antigen present on the surface of the schistosomulum of Schistosoma mansoni. Molecular and Biochemical Parasitology 1985;17(1): 105-114.

[73]] Balloul JM, Grzych JM, Pierce RJ, Capron A. A purified 28,000 dalton protein from Schistosoma mansoni adult worms protects rats and mice against experimental schistosomiasis. Journal of Immunology 1987;138(10): 3448-3453.

[74] Nutten S, Papin JP, Woerly G, Dunne DW, MacGregor J, Trottein F, Capron M. Selectin and Lewis(x) are required as co-receptors in antibody-dependent cell-mediated cytotoxicity of human eosinophils to Schistosoma mansoni schistosomula. European Journal of Immunology 1999;29(3): 799-808.

[75] Moser G, Sher A. Studies of the antibody-dependent killing of schistosomula of Schistosoma mansoni employing haptenic target antigens. II. In vitro killing of TNP-schistosomula by human eosinophils and neutrophils. Journal of Immunology 1981;126(3): 1025-1029.

[76] Lehn M, Chiang CP, Remold HG, Swafford JR, Caulfield JP. Freshly isolated and cultured human monocytes obtained by plasmapheresis kill schistosomula of Schistosoma mansoni. American Journal of Pathology 1991;139(2): 399-411.

[77] Kusel JR, Gordon JF. Biophysical studies of the schistosome surface and their relevance to its properties under immune and drug attack. Parasite Immunology 1989;11(5): 431-451.

[78] Gobert GN, Chai M, McManus DP. Biology of the schistosome lung-stage schistosomulum. Parasitology 2007;134(Pt 4): 453-460.

[79] Crabtree JE, Wilson RA. Schistosoma mansoni: a scanning electron microscope study of the developing schistosomulum. Parasitology 1980;81(Pt 3): 553-564.

[80] Krautz-Peterson G, Camargo S, Huggel K, Verrey F, Shoemaker CB, Skelly PJ. Amino acid transport in schistosomes: Characterization of the permease heavy chain SPRM1hc. Journal of Biological Chemistry 2007;282(30): 21767-21775.

[81] Krautz-Peterson G, Simoes M, Faghiri Z, Ndegwa D, Oliveira G, Shoemaker CB, Skelly PJ. Suppressing glucose transporter gene expression in schistosomes impairs parasite feeding and decreases survival in the mammalian host. PLoS Pathogens 2010;6(6): e1000932.

[82] Da'dara A, Krautz-Peterson G, Faghiri Z, Skelly PJ. Metabolite movement across the schistosome surface. Journal of Helminthology 2012;86(2): 141-147.

[83] Dean DA. Decreased binding of cytotoxic antibody by developing Schistosoma mansoni. Evidence for a surface change independent of host antigen adsorption and membrane turnover. Journal of Parasitolology 1977;63(3): 418-426.

[84] Dessein A, Samuelson JC, Butterworth AE, Hogan M, Sherry BA, Vadas MA, David JR. Immune evasion by Schistosoma mansoni: loss of susceptibility to antibody or complement-dependent eosinophil attack by schistosomula cultured in medium free of macromolecules. Parasitology 1981;82(3): 357-374.

[85] McLaren DJ, Terry RJ. The protective role of acquired host antigens during schistosome maturation. Parasite Immunology 1982; 4(2): 129-148.

[86] Pearce EJ, Basch PF, Sher A. Evidence that the reduced surface antigenicity of developing Schistosoma mansoni schistosomula is due to antigen shedding rather than host molecule acquisition. Parasite Immunology 1986;8 (1): 79-94.

[87] Foley M, MacGregor AN, Kusel JR, Garland PB, Downie T, Moore I. The lateral diffusion of lipid probes in the surface membrane of Schistosoma mansoni. Journal of Cell Biology 1986;103(3): 807-818.

[88] Chiang C-P, Caulfield JP. Human lipoprotein binding to schistosomula of Schistosoma mansoni. Displacement by polyanions, parasite antigen masking, and persistence in young larvae. American Journal of Pathology 1989:135(6): 1015-1024.

[89] Kusel JR, Al-Adhami BH, Doenhoff MJ. The schistosome in the mammalian host: understanding the mechanisms of adaptation. Parasitology 2007;134(Pt 11): 1477-1526

[90] Tallima H, El Ridi R. Schistosoma mansoni glyceraldehyde 3-phosphate dehydrogenase is a lung-stage schistosomula surface membrane antigen. Folia Parasitology (Praha) 2008;55(3): 180-186.

[91] Skelly PJ, Wilson RA. Making sense of the schistosome surface. Advances in Parasitology 2006;63: 185-284.

[92] El Ridi R, Mohamed SH, Tallima H. Incubation of Schistosoma mansoni lung-stage schistosomula in corn oil exposes their surface membrane antigenic specificities. Journal of Parasitology 2003;89(5): 1064-1067.

[93] El Ridi R, Tallima H, Mohamed SH, Montash M. Depletion of Schistosoma mansoni lung-stage schistosomula cholesterol by methyl-beta-cyclodextrin dramatically increases specific antibody binding to surface membrane antigens. Journal of Parasitology 2004;90(4): 727-732.

[94] Tallima H, El Ridi R. Methyl-beta-cyclodextrin treatment and filipin staining reveal the role of cholesterol in surface membrane antigen sequestration of Schistosoma mansoni and S. haematobium lung-stage larvae. Journal of Parasitology 2005;91(3): 720-725.

[95] Tallima H, Salah M, El-Ridi R. In vitro and in vivo effects of unsaturated fatty acids on Schistosoma mansoni and S. haematobium lung-stage larvae. Journal of Parasitology 2005;91(5): 1094-1102.

[96] El Ridi R, Tallima H. Equilibrium in lung schistosomula sphingomyelin breakdown and biosynthesis allows very small molecules, but not antibody, to access proteins at the host-parasite interface. Journal of Parasitology 2006;92(4): 730-737.

[97] Tallima H, Hamada M, El Ridi R. Evaluation of cholesterol content and impact on antigen exposure in the outer lipid bilayer of adult schistosomes. Parasitology 2007;134(Pt 12): 1775-1783.

[98] Berriman M, Haas BJ, LoVerde PT, Wilson RA, Dillon GP, Cerqueira GC, Mashiyama ST, Al-Lazikani B, Andrade LF, Ashton PD, Aslett MA, Bartholomeu DC, Blandin G, Caffrey CR, Coghlan A, Coulson R, Day TA, Delcher A, DeMarco R, Djikeng A, Eyre T, Gamble JA, Ghedin E, Gu Y, Hertz-Fowler C, Hirai H, Hirai Y, Houston R, Ivens A, Johnston DA, Lacerda D, Macedo CD, McVeigh P, Ning Z, Oliveira G, Overington JP, Parkhill J, Pertea M, Pierce RJ, Protasio AV, Quail MA, Rajandream MA, Rogers J, Sajid M, Salzberg SL, Stanke M, Tivey AR, White O, Williams DL, Wortman J, Wu W, Zamanian M, Zerlotini A, Fraser-Liggett CM, Barrell BG, El-Sayed NM. The genome of the blood fluke Schistosoma mansoni. Nature 2009;460(7253): 352-358.

[99] Young ND, Jex AR, Li B, Liu S, Yang L, Xiong Z, Li Y, Cantacessi C, Hall RS, Xu X, Chen F, Wu X, Zerlotini A, Oliveira G, Hofmann A, Zhang G, Fang X, Kang Y, Campbell BE, Loukas A, Ranganathan S, Rollinson D, Rinaldi G, Brindley PJ, Yang H, Wang J, Wang J, Gasser RB. Whole-genome sequence of Schistosoma haematobium. Nature Genetics 2012;44(2): 221-225.

[100] Tallima H, Al-Halbosiy MF, El Ridi R. Enzymatic activity and immunolocalization of Schistosoma mansoni and Schistosoma haematobium neutral sphingomyelinase. Molecular and Biochemical Parasitology 2011;178(1): 23-28.

[101] El Ridi R, Aboueldahab M, Tallima H, Salah M, Mahana N, Fawzi S, Mohamed SH, Fahmy OM. In vitro and in vivo activities of arachidonic acid against Schistosoma mansoni and Schistosoma haematobium. Antimicrobial Agents and Chemotherapy 2010;54(8): 3383-3389.

[102] El Ridi R, Tallima H, Salah M, Aboueldahab M, Fahmy OM, Al-Halbosiy MF, Mahmoud SS. Efficacy and mechanism of action of arachidonic acid in the treatment of hamsters infected with Schistosoma mansoni or Schistosoma haematobium. International Journal of Antimicrobial Agents 2012;39(3): 232-239.

[103] El Ridi RAF, Tallima HA-M. Novel therapeutic and prevention approaches for schistosomiasis. Journal of Advanced Research 2012 (in press). http://dx.doi.org/10.1016/j.jare.2012.05.002

[104] Skelly P. Fighting killer worms. Scientific American 2008;298(5): 94-99

[105] Knudsen GM, Medzihradszky KF, Lim KC, Hansell E, McKerrow JH. Proteomic analysis of Schistosoma mansoni cercarial secretions. Molecular and Cellular Proteomics 2005;4(12):1862-1875.

[106] Curwen RS, Ashton PD, Sundaralingam S, Wilson RA. Identification of novel proteases and immunomodulators in the secretions of schistosome cercariae that facilitate host entry. Molecular and Cellular Proteomics 2006;5(5): 835-844.

[107] Jang-Lee J, Curwen RS, Ashton PD, Tissot B, Mathieson W, Panico M, Dell A, Wilson RA, Haslam SM. Glycomics analysis of Schistosoma mansoni egg and cercarial secretions. Molecular and Cellular Proteomics 2007;6(9): 1485-1499.

[108] Hansell E, Braschi S, Medzihradszky KF, Sajid M, Debnath M, Ingram J, Lim KC, McKerrow JH. Proteomic analysis of skin invasion by blood fluke larvae. PLoS Neglected Tropical Diseases 2008; 2(7): e262.

[109] Liu F, Cui SJ, Hu W, Feng Z, Wang ZQ, Han ZG. Excretory/secretory proteome of the adult developmental stage of human blood fluke, Schistosoma japonicum. Molecular and Cellular Proteomics 2009;8(6): 1236-1251.

[110] El Ridi R, Tallima H. Schistosoma mansoni ex vivo lung-stage larvae excretory-secretory antigens as vaccine candidates against schistosomiasis. Vaccine 2009;27(5): 666-673.

[111] Liao Q, Yuan X, Xiao H, Liu C, Lv Z, Zhao Y, Wu Z. Identifying Schistosoma japonicum excretory/secretory proteins and their interactions with host immune system. PLoS One 2011;6(8): e23786.

[112] Mountford AP, Trottein F. Schistosomes in the skin: a balance between immune priming and regulation. Trends in Parasitology 2004;20(5): 221-226.

[113] Jenkins SJ, Hewitson JP, Ferret-Bernard S, Mountford AP. Schistosome larvae stimulate macrophage cytokine production through TLR4-dependent and -independent pathways. International Immunology 2005;17(11): 1409-1418.

[114] Jenkins SJ, Hewitson JP, Jenkins GR, Mountford AP. Modulation of the host's immune response by schistosome larvae. Parasite Immunology 2005;27(10-11): 385-393.

[115] Jenkins SJ, Mountford AP. Dendritic cells activated with products released by schistosome larvae drive Th2-type immune responses, which can be inhibited by manipulation of CD40 costimulation. Infection and Immunity 2005;73(1): 395-402.

[116] Paveley RA, Aynsley SA, Turner JD, Bourke CD, Jenkins SJ, Cook PC, Martinez-Pomares L, Mountford AP. The Mannose Receptor (CD206) is an important pattern recognition receptor (PRR) in the detection of the infective stage of the helminth Schistosoma mansoni and modulates IFNγ production. International Journal for Parasitology 2011;41(13-14): 1335-1345.

[117] Robinson MW, Hutchinson AT, Donnelly S, Dalton JP. Worm secretory molecules are causing alarm. Trends in Parasitology 2010;26(8): 371-372.

[118] Coulson PS. The radiation-attenuated vaccine against schistosomes in animal models: paradigm for a human vaccine? Advances in Parasitology 1997;39: 271-336.

[119] Dale DC, Boxer L, Liles WC. The phagocytes: neutrophils and monocytes. Blood 2008; 112(4): 935-945.

[120] Ahmed SF, Oswald IP, Caspar P, Hieny S, Keefer L, Sher A, James SL. Developmental differences determine larval susceptibility to nitric oxide-mediated killing in a murine model of vaccination against Schistosoma mansoni. Infection and Immunity 1997;65(1): 219-226.

[121] Coulson PS, Smythies LE, Betts C, Mabbott NA, Sternberg JM, Wei XG, Liew FY, Wilson RA. Nitric oxide produced in the lungs of mice immunized with the radiation-attenuated schistosome vaccine is not the major agent causing challenge parasite elimination. Immunology 1998; 93(1);55-63.

[122] Medina E. Neutrophil extracellular traps: a strategic tactic to defeat pathogens with potential consequences for the host. Journal of Innate Immunity 2009;1(3): 176-180.

[123] Menegazzi R, Decleva E, Dri P. Killing by neutrophil extracellular traps: fact or folklore? Blood 2012;119(5): 1214-1216.

[124] Ackerman SJ, Gleich GJ, Loegering DA, Richardson BA, Butterworth AE. Comparative toxicity of purified human eosinophil granule cationic proteins for schistosomula of Schistosoma mansoni. American Journal of Tropical Medicine and Hygiene 1985;34(4): 735-745.

[125] Blanchard C, Rothenberg ME. Biology of the eosinophil. Advances in Immunology 2009;101: 81-121.

[126] Schroeder JT. Basophils beyond effector cells of allergic inflammation. Advances in Immunology 2009;101: 123-161.

[127] Anderson S, Shires VL, Wilson RA, Mountford AP. In the absence of IL-12, the induction of Th1-mediated protective immunity by the attenuated schistosome vaccine is impaired, revealing an alternative pathway with Th2-type characteristics. European Journal of Immunology 1998;28(9): 2827-2838.

[128] Jankovic D, Wynn TA, Kullberg MC, Hieny S, Caspar P, James S, Cheever AW, Sher A. Optimal vaccination against Schistosoma mansoni requires the induction of both B cell- and IFN-gamma-dependent effector mechanisms. Journal of Immunology 1999;162(1): 345-351.

[129] Mountford AP, Hogg KG, Coulson PS, Brombacher F. Signaling via interleukin-4 receptor alpha chain is required for successful vaccination against schistosomiasis in BALB/c mice. Infection and Immunity 2001;69(1): 228-236.

[130] Hewitson JP, Hamblin PA, Mountford AP. Immunity induced by the radiation-attenuated schistosome vaccine. Parasite Immunology 2005;27(7-8): 271-280.

[131] Cêtre C, Cocude C, Pierrot C, Godin C, Capron A, Capron M, Khalife J. In vivo expression of cytokine mRNA in rats infected with Schistosoma mansoni. Parasite Immunology 1998;20(3): 135-142.

[132] Cêtre C, Pierrot C, Cocude C, Lafitte S, Capron A, Capron M, Khalife J. Profiles of Th1 and Th2 cytokines after primary and secondary infection by Schistosoma mansoni in the semipermissive rat host. Infection and Immunity1999;67(6): 2713-2719.

[133] Fallon PG, Gibbons J, Vervenne RA, Richardson EJ, Fulford AJ, Kiarie S, Sturrock RF, Coulson PS, Deelder AM, Langermans JA, Thomas AW, Dunne DW. Juvenile rhesus monkeys have lower type 2 cytokine responses than adults after primary infection with Schistosoma mansoni. Journal of Infectious Diseases 2003;187(6): 939-945.

[134] Ganley-Leal LM, Mwinzi PN, Cetre-Sossah CB, Andove J, Hightower AW, Karanja DM, Colley DG, Secor WE. Correlation between eosinophils and protection against reinfection with Schistosoma mansoni and the effect of human immunodeficiency virus type 1 coinfection in humans. Infection and Immunity 2006;74(4): 2169-2176.

[135] Black CL, Mwinzi PN, Muok EM, Abudho B, Fitzsimmons CM, Dunne DW, Karanja DM, Secor WE, Colley DG. Influence of exposure history on the immunology and development of resistance to human Schistosomiasis mansoni. PLoS Neglected Tropical Diseases 2010; 23;4(3): e637.

[136] Figueiredo JP, Oliveira RR, Cardoso LS, Barnes KC, Grant AV, Carvalho EM, Araujo MI. Adult worm-specific IgE/IgG4 balance is associated with low infection levels of Schistosoma mansoni in an endemic area. Parasite Immunology 2012 (in press). doi: 10.1111/pim.12001

[137] El Ridi R, Tallima H. Adjuvant selection for vaccination against murine schistosomiasis. Scandinavian Journal of Immunology 2012; in press. DOI: 10.1111/j. 1365-3083.2012.02768.x

[138] El Ridi R, Tallima H. Vaccine-induced protection against murine schistosomiasis mansoni with larval excretory-secretory antigens and papain or type-2 cytokines. Journal of Parasitology 2012; in press. DOI: http://dx.doi.org/10.1645/GE-3186.1